warm, witty and very, very wise – the perfect
antidote to all those po-faced pregnancy books.
As a fellow Geriatric mother I found myself constantly
laughing and nodding along in agreement'
Imogen Edwards-Jones

Cari Rosen worked for many years as a
TV producer before becoming a mum for the first
time at 43. Her experience as a 'midlife mum'
formed the basis of her popular column in the
Jewish Chronicle. This is her first book.
www.carirosen.com

For my girl

THE SECRET DIARY OF A NEW MUM (AGED 43¼)

CARI ROSEN

Vermilion
LONDON

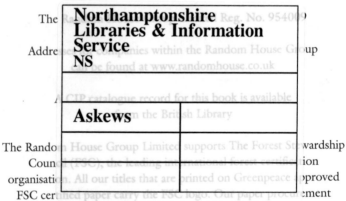

The Ra_____ Reg. No. 954009

Addre_____nies within the Random House Group
___ be found at www.randomhouse.co.uk

A CIP catalogue record for this book is available
_____ the British Library

Northamptonshire Libraries & Information Service NS

Askews

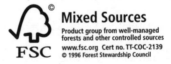

Mixed Sources
Product group from well-managed
forests and other controlled sources
www.fsc.org Cert no. TT-COC-2139
© 1996 Forest Stewardship Council
FSC

Designed and set by seagulls.net

Printed in the UK by CPI Mackays, Chatham, ME5 8TD

ISBN 9780091935658

To buy books by your favourite authors and register for offers visit
www.rbooks.co.uk

CONTENTS

Preface *1*

Chapter 1: Fat and 40 *3*

Chapter 2: Happy Birth-day *41*

Chapter 3: 0–3 Months *61*

Chapter 4: 3–6 Months *93*

Chapter 5: 6–9 Months *113*

Chapter 6: 9–12 Months *137*

Chapter 7: 12–18 Months *157*

Chapter 8: 18–24 Months *193*

Chapter 9: Turning Two *225*

Epilogue *241*

Acknowledgments *249*

PREFACE

I am sitting in the toilet at work. Outside the cubicle two girls are talking about a gig they have been to the night before.

'Amazing, wasn't it?'

'Yeah – but it was ruined by this old couple in front of us snogging all night.'

'How old?'

'God – really old. About 35.'

'That's disgusting … '

I am trying not to cry.

I am clutching a Superdrug carrier bag full of newly purchased pregnancy tests. Best to wait till I get home, I think. Then – no, will try now. Get it over with.

Fumble with packet, pee on stick, wait the required 30 seconds – knowing that it will be disappointment once again.

But it is blue. It is blue. I am 42 years old and pregnant. I am apparently too old to kiss in public, but not too old to have a baby.

I cannot stop shaking. I burst into tears, then am forced to remain in the cubicle for another half hour until I am fit to be seen in public.

Ring husband from car park. He is in a meeting. I cry some more. He cries too. Apologises to everyone in the meeting …

CHAPTER 1

FAT AND 40

According to the midwife, I am a geriatric mother. Well, technically, I am a geriatric Jewish mother, which means not only am I (apparently) terribly old, but I also worry. A lot. Though on the plus side, I do make fabulous chicken soup.

The term 'geriatric mother' instantly conjures up visions of old dears on Zimmer frames, lilac rinses and canasta every Tuesday. True, I don't quite fit this stereotype – though give me 30 years and a chance to brush up on my card skills, and there's a strong chance I will be forced to eat my words.

But for now, suffice to say that I am very delighted at the prospect of being a new mum – and rather less than delighted to hear that I am a fair way past my prime.

Indeed, any illusions I may have about clinging on to the last vestiges of youth are shattered at the very start of my gestational journey when I leaf through my notes and see the term 'elderly primigravida' used with gay abandon throughout.

Why not shout from the rooftops, 'I am old, I am old. I should be knitting for my grandchildren?'

But aside from the technicality that I can't knit, the fact remains that I am sitting here in my own right, in the pregnancy wing of a busy London hospital. In all my 40-something glory, I am huffing and puffing among mothers-to-be who are young enough to be my daughters, while the medical staff puzzle over whether to admit me to maternity or geriatrics.

It doesn't help that the patient sitting next to me looks like a child herself. I sneak a peek at her folder and the birth date emblazoned on the front confirms that she was born in 1992. A quick tally on fingers and thumbs (maths never having been my strong point) reveals she is indeed just 16 and that I am, therefore, almost 27 years older than she is. *Twenty-seven* years.

It is a very long time since I was 16 and in the intervening years I have done O levels (for that is what they were in my day), A levels and a degree. I have been a Mod and a Punk and a New Romantic (not necessarily in that order). I have had a career. Bought two flats (not at the same time). Done three parachute jumps. Earned a living. Filled in tax returns. And I've killed one goldfish and an embarrassingly large number of house plants.

And yet, here in this room full of posters reminding us to wash our hands and avoid dog faeces, all this life experience counts for nothing. Sitting here, we are on a par, she and I. In the same boat – the Good Ship Stretch Mark – clutching our still-warm urine samples and waiting to be called. We both have puffy ankles and bulging bellies. We are both nurturing a new life within. It's just that I'm old enough to be her mother (yes, and by this token grandmother – yikes – to her child). Plus, I'm plainly also a lot less willing to bare my bump to the world by wearing skimpy Lycra crop tops and hip-hugging flares in the dead of winter. Or any other season, come to that.

An 'elderly prim' I might be, but I still find it strange to be so clearly defined by my age. I have obviously let the last few birthdays wash over me without noticing exactly how often they came around. And it's not as though I actually set out to be an older mum (or wear elasticated-waist trousers for that matter), but it would appear that it has just sort of happened this way.

Story after story in certain newspapers tell me I must be (among other things) a selfish workaholic who has given her best years to her career and now wants to have it all. But this could not be further from the truth.

Yes, I have loved my job (travelling the world to interview the likes of Sting, Yoko Ono and the Goombay Dance Band – what's not to like?). It is true that I have worked hard and achieved what I wanted to – but certainly not to the exclusion of all else. My evenings, weekends and holidays have been as filled with friends, relationships and fun as anyone else's. Hell, I've even found the time to do a City & Guilds in ceramics.

And indeed, this is not the first opportunity that I have been offered to procreate; it is simply the first one that has not had me running for the hills at the realisation that accepting would leave me irrevocably tied to someone I don't really want to spend the rest of my life with (but thank you for asking). It was not until my late 30s that I had the good fortune to meet the person I actually *did* want to start a family with. And so it was that circumstance (including a major gynae op), not choice, dictated that for me life – or at least new life – really does begin at 40.

Thankfully, I am not alone in this. Sure, half my friends did their childbearing years ago and are now at the stage of panicking about puberty and tearing their hair out over secondary-school choices and Ofsted reports. But the rest are only getting started now, and are thus also on the first leg of their voyage into the world of nappies, *Night Garden* and nipple shields.

Like me, these women do not conform to the media stereotypes and almost all say that finding the right part-ner is their reason for delay. As one close friend confides: 'It's not ideal – but what could I do? It took me bloody ages to find the right man – or indeed any man that would have me.'

And if Mr Right proves elusive, unreliable or unwill-ing, as he has done for a fair number of women of my acquaintance, it's a stark choice. Give up on the dream? Or grab yourself some sperm?

Let's face facts: in Britain alone, 26,419 women in their 40s had babies in 2008 – a figure that has doubled in just a decade and doesn't take into account the many thousands of women in their mid- to late 30s who also gave birth – and who are also classed as 'older mums'. (An additional 116,220 in case you were wondering, which, when you tot it all up, means that almost a fifth of all babies born that year were to mums aged 35 plus.)

It is, therefore, possibly unwise for anyone to assume that each and every one of these tens of thousands of women must be either a 'career-crazed power freak' (a phrase that particularly charmed me on one radio phone-in) or 'a minger who can't get a husband' (overheard in a local park).

But whatever the many and varied reasons for our delay, we quadragenarians still appear to be considered practically prehistoric in reproductive terms. It's a bit of a bombshell to have this spelled out quite so clearly as I've never really felt that old before. But then delusion is a wonderful thing …

Truth be told, it came as something of a shock to realise that somehow, when I wasn't looking, my 40s had managed to sneak up from behind, bestowing upon me a couple of extra dress sizes that I really couldn't remember ordering and enough grey hairs for my mother to suggest the immediate purchase of a job lot of Garnier Nutrisse.

Suddenly I realised that apparently it was *me* who the papers were shouting at, with their constant reminders that once you're over 35 your chances of giving birth start to decline at an alarming rate.

My natural instinct was to yell back at them very loudly, 'I know, I know. It's not like I am doing this on purpose.' Though I soon discovered that actually doing that could lead to a lifetime ban from the local newsagent – the cause of some embarrassment, not to mention great inconvenience.

But those headlines kept on coming … Womph – a story about another woman who had left it too late. Eek

– a front-page splash warning that my fertility had actually been in freefall since my late 20s, not my mid-30s as I had previously thought.

The articles seemed to appear with such frequency that I was half-expecting a town crier to greet me outside Tesco yelling, 'Oyez, oyez, buy your eggs here because the ones you've got are no use to anyone.'

The outlook was frosty doom and gloom on every corner, and everything I could find to read on making babies as an 'older' mum led me to believe that heading down the IVF clinic was most likely my only option.

And so it came as a pleasant surprise to discover that my reproductive bits were actually working very nicely, thank you, and I was pregnant within weeks.

But on that occasion our joy was short lived. I had only just got over the shock of how quickly my ancient ovaries had sprung into action when an early scan failed to find a heartbeat. We had to wait two more weeks until we knew for sure, but in our hearts we knew that our little 'Dot' was not to be. This turned out to be 'one of those things', entirely unrelated to my age. Everyone at the hospital was unfailingly kind throughout the process – though elsewhere people trotted out statistics about miscarriage rates shooting up to one in every two pregnancies once you hit the big 4–0. Not for the first time,

I wondered whether motherhood really might be an impossible dream.

And then I met one doctor who said it was a miracle I got pregnant at all at my age and warned me not to count on it happening again. When I told him that actually I knew loads of women who had had babies in their 40s he told me that those were just the ones you hear about. Most are not successful.

I returned home devastated. But then bloody-mindedness set in. Of course, medically speaking, the doctor may have been right – but that was not going to stop me trying to prove him wrong. I read up on the figures that told me that at 40 my fertility rate was 20 per cent and that it would drop to one per cent at the age of 45. But I also figured that if so many people I knew had managed to get themselves up the duff despite these odds, there had to be at least a glimmer of hope – and I was going to grasp it with both hands, wrestle it to the floor and hide it under the bed for as long as I possibly could.

I followed all the traditionally recommended routes to the letter and took my folic acid with unerring regularity – but encouragement came from an unexpected source. A friend (not exactly a youngster herself at 39) announced that she was with child. And after three failed

IVFs it was a natural conception. 'It must be because my hubby went out for a curry that night,' she joked.

I didn't pay much attention to this until another friend announced that she was pregnant too. She'd already told us that IVF was her only hope – a slim one at that – but chatting to the delighted mum-to-be I discovered that the night before the procedure her husband had also been tucking into a tikka. Same restaurant. Same table. And bingo ...

I grabbed my diary, kept tabs on my cycle and worked out the next date I was most likely to conceive. Then, on the evening in question, my husband was inducted into the 'curry club'. There were the inevitable jokes about him heading home for a bit of 'argy bhaji' and complex arrangements with trains back from a meeting up North on my part, but it turned out to be worth the hassle. Call it korma, karma or even wishful thinking, but it worked.

Yes, yes, it may well be that the acupuncture, the two rounds of Clomid and the judicious use of ovulation sticks had something to do with it – but no matter.

... And so here I am now, six months after our first visit – back in the early pregnancy unit and sick with nerves before my scan.

The same room, the same staff, the same anxious search for a sign of life. The minutes pass and we prepare ourselves for the worst. Just as we start to think that all is lost, there it is. A teeny tiny pinprick flickering in the centre of the screen. I burst into tears of relief and cry for the rest of the day.

I decide that I do not want to tell anyone our news until we reach the three-month stage. But soon I discover it is very hard to keep a secret when you cannot even open the fridge without retching. It is autumn – a disaster in culinary terms, as soon my open-plan office is filled with people sipping soup for lunch, with every whiff of carrot and coriander, tomato and basil or spicy lentil sending me heaving to seek refuge in the car park.

Most of the time, the very thought of food makes me gag. One day, I become convinced that the only thing I can possibly stomach is a Findus French Bread Pizza. I drive round and round north London until I find one (harder than you might think). I stick it in the oven, take just one bite, then do all I can to avoid being within 300 yards of one for the rest of my gestation (easier than you might think). It's a similar situation with Super Noodles.

A few weeks on and I am spending eight hours a day in an edit suite where it is difficult to disguise the fact that I am living on dry bread and grapes. I invent stomach bugs, reactions to antibiotics, anything I can think of to distract my colleagues from the truth. Perhaps I over-egg the pudding, for soon I have a reputation as a hypochondriac and a malingerer.

At home, I discover that one way to cope is to keep a bowl of dry cornflakes by the bed. But night-time nausea is not terribly romantic and my husband complains that my constant crunching is keeping him awake. And so I suck my cereal, slowly, slowly. By the time I have finished I have had no sleep at all – but at least marital harmony is restored.

In the early stages of my pregnancy, my geriatric status affords me fortnightly scans, though other than that I begin to forget about my age. But at 11 weeks, all that changes. A long weekend at work, a telephone call bringing bad news – and stomach cramps so bad that I can barely stand. At 4am, I am in A&E, doubled up in pain and convinced that it is all over. And this is the moment when it hits me; this could very well be my last-chance saloon. How many times can I go through this? How many times can we try again before the biological clock runs out of juice? 'Please, little Bean, hang on in there,' I whisper.

Whether fortune is smiling upon us, or whether my child is as bloody-minded as its mother I do not know, but a scan shows that all is well.

At 12 weeks I am offered a combined test to assess the risk of Downs and other abnormalities. Regardless of how fit and healthy the mum is, this is where age really comes into play: at under 25 your risk starts out at around one in 1,500, at 35 it's one in 300 and at 45 it soars to one in 22.

My overall result comes back at one in 750, 'as good as it can be for your age,' the doctor tells me. But now I have started to panic about all the other things that might go wrong. My husband bans me from reading baby books because the bad bits leap out at me every time I turn a page. Instead, each night, he reads me carefully selected passages ensuring he picks out nothing more daunting than cradle cap or cravings.

I wonder if it's an age thing: am I worrying more because I am older? But apparently not. Almost everyone else I ask is calm and serene throughout, and the few who are uneasy describe themselves as worriers in general – women who have sleepless nights about whether they have enough milk in the fridge for breakfast or clean socks for work …

... which then makes me worry about whether there is indeed enough milk in the fridge for breakfast and deeply concerned about the state of my sock drawer on top of all the other things as well.

I am advised against an amnio, partly because the risk of miscarriage outweighs the odds of abnormality – but mainly because my previous test results do not warrant an invasive procedure.

Because I am older I am offered consultant-led care, and every time I have a hospital appointment I get to see a wonderful obstetrician who assuages each new set of worries with calm and patience.

'No, no, the nose doesn't look squashy at all on the scan ... Yes, I am absolutely sure it's fine to go on a plane if you want to ... Yes, it is true that some women get enlarged and swollen varicose veins in their vagina while they are pregnant, but I don't think you need to worry too much about that ... Absolutely, you can raise your arms above your head without the baby choking on its umbilical cord ... And yes, I do advise women to avoid scuba diving if they can.'

(For reference, I have never actually been scuba diving and nor do I intend to start – particularly given the fact I have a long-standing terror of any form of seaweed that is not wrapped around a piece of sushi –

but it's good to know where I stand in case the need should arise at any point over the next few months …)*

Slowly, I start to share my news. Family and friends are thrilled. But as well as the 'fabs' and the 'wows' and the 'over the moons' I also get the odd 'Blimey' and 'Nappies at your age? You must be mad!' And despite my carefully selected baggies, it seems my weight gain has not gone as unnoticed at work as I'd thought.

'Guess what, everyone?' yells my boss to the crowded office. 'She's not fat after all. She's pregnant!'

And I am not overjoyed to have my belly described as a 'comedy bump' in the middle of a meeting.

But actually, I find my baby bump strangely liberating. There's no more sucking in my stomach for special occasions – now I am out and proud, albeit struggling to find clothes to accommodate my newly curvaceous form.

In an institution renowned for its purveyance of finery to the mother-to-be I head off to the changing

---

* In fact, I have a text-book pregnancy during which everything does exactly what it is meant to do. And, with a trusty bottle of Gaviscon by my side at all times, I bloom and glow throughout my second and third trimesters.

room to try on a couple of tops, and there I discover that someone has left their backpack behind. So while I strip off and start grappling with the various layers of Lycra that every outfit appears to involve, I dispatch my husband to track down an assistant and hand it in, lest the owner returns to collect it.

He reappears soon after, red-faced, explaining that the backpack is, in fact, a prosthetic 'bump', designed to give women in the earlier stages of pregnancy an idea of how an outfit might look when they have reached the size of a three-seater sofa.

Working on the basis of 'when in Rome', I give it a go myself – although actually getting the damned thing on turns out to be fractionally more testing than achieving a first-class honours degree in astrophysics. It is at the point when I have wrestled the thing to the floor in a bid to stop it strangling me and am lying alongside it prostrate, weeping with laughter in full view of the entire emporium that my husband takes charge and removes me to a shopping centre up the road.

There, I try over-the-bump trousers – they fall down constantly. I try under-the-bump trousers. They too fall down constantly. I cannot figure out where to put a belt so that it doesn't dig into my tummy – and so am resigned to the fact that for months on end I'll be forced to hitch myself up every time I take more than two steps at a time. It's not a great look.

My breasts, which, to be fair, were not exactly concave beforehand (I recall my husband once asking whether 'F' stood for 'flipping enormous' as we perused the wares in one lingerie store) are now the size of watermelons and weigh approximately six stone each. I am not overly chuffed to discover that this fact is now considered a suitable topic for dinner-party discussion.

It is also impossible to get comfortable in bed. I can no longer sleep on my stomach, partly for fear that I will look like an upended turtle, but mainly because I don't want to squash the poor child before it's even here. I have never been able to sleep on my back, and when I lie on my side everything seems to be getting in the way of everything else. I am forced to wear more underwear and upholstery at night than I do during the day, but with the baby now asserting its prowess as a footballer, any cushioning and corsetry is largely irrelevant.

I find that I am also spending a slightly unreasonable amount of time contemplating my navel. This is not because I don't have better things to do, but because for as long as I can remember I have had something of a belly-button phobia. I will own that on a day-to-day basis this is not an enormous issue, given that for the majority of the time it is hidden under a T-shirt and therefore easy to ignore. But suddenly pregnancy has put its 'innie' status in jeopardy and the very idea of an 'outie' fills me with (disproportionate) revulsion.

Each evening, I've been requesting that my husband checks how much shallower it is than the night before. And each evening he rolls his eyes and assures me that there's still a long way to go. He's right, as it happens, but this does not stop me fixating on the waistline of every other pregnant woman I meet and assessing the probability.

Then there are stretch marks. A friend has suggested that the best way to avoid them is to rub Bio Oil into the bump on a regular basis. I mention this to my husband who duly comes home with a bottle of Baby Bio. It is not that I do not appreciate his contribution – just that I was aiming for suppleness of skin, rather than greener leaves and vibrant flowers.

Where I live, and within my own circle of friends and colleagues, it seems to be no rarity to be fecund and 40 and I feel very fortunate to be among people who have seen it all before. But even in this great metropolis, others are not so lucky. My friend Sophie informs me that when people saw she was pregnant they assumed that:

a) it was her second or third baby
b) she'd had IVF or AI
c) she was just really, really fat
d) she and her husband had been trying unsuc-
   cessfully for years *or*
e) she had killed husbands one, two and three
   before meeting husband number four who
   was able to father a child with her.

Another friend relates how at her last antenatal appointment her midwife called her *ancient*! While Kate, a GP
who between the ages of 36 and 45 has had four kids,
found that even being a medic herself didn't help stop
people from reacting inappropriately with comments
like, 'You are a doctor, you should know how to stop
this happening!'

One chum (38) adds, 'I didn't really think about my
age at all – and it was only a load of comments about me
being "an older mother" that brought it to my attention.

Actually it's a bit of a shock to realise that I'm now
considered to be a grown-up. After all, I have never
owned a pedestal mat, I still live in fear that I will incur
my mother's wrath when I stay over and leave the valance
more than 0.1mm adrift of its "natural drop" – and it's
still a source of some incredulity that I now possess a
dinner service where everything matches.'

Living in this multimedia age, an era in which we are assailed on all sides by TV and radio and newspapers and the Internet ... well, sometimes it is hard to know what to think. Conflicting opinion is at every turn.

One minute, for example, the headlines are screaming that butter 'gives us heart attacks' and we should all eat marg instead. Then, the next minute, marg is 'carcinogenic', so we all go back to butter ... And it seems that older motherhood is no different (other than the fact that you can't get it in your online Tesco shop).

Panic! A piece in the paper is telling us that babies born to older mums are more likely to have growth problems in the womb (something about our placentas not developing as efficiently, but I am too flustered to take in much of the detail, other than the fact that we are one and a half times more likely to run into this than younger mums). Then relief! A magazine article is now proclaiming that mid-life motherhood confers a multitude of benefits.

And although I know it is a big mistake on my part to trawl the Internet to try to find out what these are, I learn:

1) Older mums are more likely to have multiple births. (Check scan – no, definitely just the one. Phew.)

2) We have a higher risk of Caesarean or stillbirth.

3) We are (according to a website I accidentally click on in search of a morale boost) sexy, sexy beasts who you can call on 0800 MID-AGE MOMMAS to satisfy any lustful urges.

But then there is a spate of sensational headlines about gestating grannies and so I take to surfing some more and reading stories about post-menopausal women in their 50s, 60s, even 70s who are popping out infants willy nilly. Hurrah – by the time I have finished, I feel like a veritable spring chicken with a whole new lease of life.

There is, after all, older motherhood and really-much-much-much-older motherhood. The former finds late-30-somethings or early-40-somethings – such as myself – eliciting the odd raised eyebrow, but not deviating too far from what nature intended. (Indeed, if nature had not intended my stomach to be swollen with child, placenta and rather too many Cadbury Creme Eggs at this stage in my life, surely my womb would not have been coerced into co-operation with quite so much ease?)

And the latter? Well, morality and mortality aside, I can see that a pensioner aiming for pregnancy is rather further from the norm and will require, without exception, an entire truckload of medical, even divine intervention.

That's not, of course, to say I have anything at all against assisted conception, but the whole senior-citizen thing? Not for me.

'I agree it's a little distasteful,' says a church-going friend as we discuss the latest documentary on procreating pensioners, 'but what people seem to forget is that it's been happening since time began and if God is okay with it, then who are we to judge?'

A quick flick through Genesis in the Old Testament and I see that she is right: ' … and Abraham fell upon his face, and laughed, and said in his heart: "Shall a child be born unto him that is a hundred years old? And shall Sarah, that is 90 years old, bear?" … And Sarah conceived, and bore Abraham a son in his old age, at the set time of which God had spoken to him.'

I feel greatly cheered. Woo hoo – good old Sarah made it through all that begetting business when she was more than double my age, though I do wonder whether she was in any fit state afterwards to push her designer off-road buggy over all that sand?

*

Back at the hospital, it's time for blood tests. Although I hate needles, I am relatively calm as I sit with my husband in the waiting room watching those before me nip in and out in a matter of moments. And then it's my turn.

I take my seat, shut my eyes and wait for the 'little scratch'. I ponder, as one does on such occasions, why they always feel the need to inform you that you'll feel said 'little scratch'? A little scratch is surely something you might expect to sustain in the course of a woodland stroll, not as the result of a 3.5 centimetre needle being rammed into your arm with force? I guess if they asked you to wait for the 'searing and agonising stab' it probably wouldn't make their job any easier. But anyway – I digress …

Roll up sleeve, make pumping motions (as directed) with fist, shut eyes, brace myself. Sharp pain and a curse that I'm surprised to find hasn't actually come from me. I gingerly raise an eyelid.

'Not a good vein,' says the nurse Sellotaping a cotton-wool ball over the wound. 'Let's try the other arm.'

Roll up sleeve, shut eyes, brace myself, pain … and … 'That's not a good vein either,' says the nurse, Sellotaping a cotton-wool ball over the wound. 'Let's try the back of your hand.'

Gingerly proffer hand, shut eyes, brace myself, pain … and … 'Oh dear,' says the nurse, Sellotaping a cotton-wool ball over this third wound. 'It's not going well for you is it?'

I am starting to panic, worrying that by the time I get out of there I will be so swathed in bandages that I'll be mistaken for the Invisible Man (but without the dark glasses). I am also concerned about where she's going to be trying next.

Reinforcements arrive and tap and poke in their search for a suitable vein. 'I'd make a lousy addict,' I joke, trying to lighten the mood, but they simply scowl at me disapprovingly and jab the needle into my other hand before I have time to close my eyes.

'Where have you been and why are you covered in pompoms?' my husband asks when I finally return to the waiting room, although I am far too traumatised to reply.

Thankfully, he is not a man to be fazed by a medical mishap. The fact that I had bronchitis and conjunctivitis – an attractive combo if ever there was one – on the day that we met would have sent many a suitor running for the hills. 'At least you've seen me at my worst,' I joked, before breaking my leg in three places just in time for our second date. And that was kind of that – as my mother wisely counselled, 'Any man who is not put off by the sight of you in those tracksuit bottoms (the only thing that would fit over the cast) for months on end is a man worth keeping.'

Indeed, I have since come to learn that he is also a man able to weather not only my decaying collection of leisure wear but my manifold peccadilloes too, including the fact that I cannot possibly sleep if a drawer is open or a cupboard door even slightly ajar. Or indeed if the 'open' end of his pillowcase faces towards me, rather than the wall (but perhaps that's one best saved for an OCD specialist).

An aunt phones to say she has just seen a new study, which shows that if you play classical music to your bump, then the baby will be a musician and if you read the classics aloud, it will be a literary genius.

On that basis, and given the amount of time we seem to spend watching *Coronation Street* or Champions League action, my husband and I can only shrug and accept the fact that our child will be a barm-cake-eating football fanatic. But hey – there are worse things in life …

Meanwhile, the days seem to crawl by and fly by all at once and suddenly it is time for the 20-week scan. Naturally, as one who worries about most things (and about having nothing else to worry about if there is actually nothing to worry about), I am worried. But all is well. The baby is upside down, happily sucking its thumb and scrutinising my knees (alas, not among my better features).

We are offered the chance to find out the sex and decline. It's not that we don't want to know (indeed, I subsequently do every online 'test' I can find – half of which inform me conclusively that I am having a boy and the other half a girl; when I joke about this to a friend she says, 'Well it could be a hermaphrodite. Didn't you read *Middlesex*?').

But the reason for my hesitation is twofold. It is partly because there are so few great surprises in life, and I want to keep this going for as long as I can. And mainly because with the baby as simply our 'Bean' I cannot visualise it in detail. If I find out whether it is a 'he' or a 'she', it will become a proper person, one that I can picture clearly – and then I will worry about it even more.

Friends – including several over 40s – find out at the first opportunity, even naming their babies before they are born. But for a nervous wreck like me, ignorance, while not quite bliss, is definitely the safest place to be.

*

It is Christmas and we attend a number of festivities, including a neighbour's drinks party, where I decline alcohol with a coy pat of my blossoming belly. Later in the evening, our host rushes to my side exclaiming (loudly), 'Oh I seeee. You are pregnant. It's just that I never thought of you as thin … '

I make a mental note to pursue a rigorous fitness campaign as soon as I have given birth. And possibly to move house.

At a festive dinner party – where, alas, I am still unable to face anything other than the now ubiquitous bread and grapes – I make a new 'friend' who adopts me as her pet and makes it her mission to keep me informed of anything and everything that might go wrong. I make the mistake of giving her my phone number.

'Helloooo,' she trills one morning, when I foolishly answer her call. 'I suddenly thought that you might not realise that your baby will probably die if you eat sushi or Stilton, so probably best to avoid until after the birth.'

I feel that to point out that millions of Japanese women give birth to healthy babies on a diet of raw fish may invoke a further diatribe from this self-appointed sage who appears to have positioned herself somewhere between Gina Ford and God. So I mutter something about only eating grapes in any case and hang up as quickly as I can.

What I do not realise is that by cutting this conversation short, I am simply giving her more time to prepare the lecture for her next call, this time focusing on the perils of pregnancy when you are past your prime: 'I thought I should warn you to try and take it easy because obviously your chances of getting high blood pressure or diabetes are so much higher than mine were. And, of course, you're way more likely to go into premature labour, so you could well end up with a low-birthweight baby which means that they will get high blood pressure too when they are older … '

I toss my mobile down the toilet and sign up for pay as you go.

A colleague suggests that meditation may be the way forward and insists that if I join her at the weekly session for mums-to-be, all my stresses and strains will vanish in an instant. Not knowing any better, I agree – which is how I find myself cross-legged on a dusty wooden floor, holding my palms aloft and chanting, 'Ommmm, ommmm'.

'Now close your eyes,' intones our instructor. 'I want you to get in touch with your vagina.'

I sneak a crafty peek, but apparently no one else in the class finds this as amusing as I do, and all appear to be communing with their nether regions without giggling or fretting over the logistics. I, however, can't even work out how to get started. As far as I am aware, my vagina is not on email, nor does it have a postal address. And as no one else in the room is shouting, 'Oy, you down there,' apparently that's not the way to go either. But it seems wrong to tap my neighbour on the shoulder and ask for enlightenment, so I just 'Omm' a bit more, then use the rest of the time to work out what I need to buy from Tesco on the way home.

A proper friend, who is relatively sane, suggests that antenatal yoga is the best way to prepare myself for the birth, so I sign up for that instead and find myself in a draughty room full of bulbous women swapping stories about haemorrhoids and incontinence (and marvelling at all the other things I never knew I should expect when I was expecting).

It's a real tonic to be among people who are also in the later stages of pregnancy and because our circumstances are the same, I blithely assume we are all about the same sort of age. Yet after a time, I notice how the others manage to nip around in nimble fashion while I discover that I need a crane and a nursing assistant to get me off the floor. It is a two-hour class, yet I excel only in the last 30 minutes – the bit where we lie on the floor wrapped in a blanket and listen to soothing and relaxing sounds. Though, to be fair, I am also pretty good at the bit after that too, where we drink herbal tea and chat over biscuits.

There is constant debate among the women I meet as to when is the best time to start a family. Some favour their 20s ('Get it all out of the way early and then they leave home and we're still young enough to travel the world and have fun,' etc. etc.). Others – the majority, certainly among those I meet – say early 30s for a whole host of reasons, including, 'It just feels right', 'I feel more settled' and 'I'm fed up with work and I want a year off'.

For those of us who come to the world of breeding rather later it can often boil down simply to 'now or never'.

One friend echoes many others when she says, 'I always thought I'd have kids when I was much younger. But it didn't work out that way. I'm just happy that I got there in the end.'

As my bump grows ever larger, I continue to make regular visits to the hospital for antenatal checks and am treated with the kind of care usually reserved for dinosaur remnants at the Natural History Museum:

unwrap carefully, allow a few chosen students to gawp in amazement at this crumbling rarity, then offer advice on preservation.

But at least I am able to use my advanced years to opportunistic advantage. As the average age for new mothers continues to rise, I have discovered a gap in the market. You may yet see me on *Dragon's Den* as the spokesperson for a new joint venture between Stannah Stairlifts and Baby Bjorn.

With a few weeks to go, we've begun our weekly ante-natal group – a course involving six Monday evenings and a lot of practice panting.

Seven couples are perched on the floor clutching pillows. There are three sets of beanbags (very comfort-able) and four sets of cushions (very uncomfortable). The competition for comfort is evident from the outset and I envisage that as the weeks go by everyone will be turning up earlier and earlier to bag the beanbags in a sort of fat-bird version of towels-on-sun-loungers.

Once again, the ages of my cohorts never crosses my mind until one classmate invites me to celebrate her 30th birthday – and I am too embarrassed to tell her I actually have a friend's 50th that night.

But at least I am not the only one to have found myself in this position.

'We were old enough to be the grandparents of most of our antenatal group,' says a chum who, at 42, is not exactly ready to be put out to pasture. 'It wasn't a major issue – just a bit of a drag socially.'

In class, it occurs to me that although I am being referred to as a 'mature' mother, I am strikingly immature in terms of my knowledge of what to do with a newborn. I dutifully write down everything I am told, from the lists of what to pack in my hospital bag to the fact that everything must be pre-washed in Fairy non-bio on pain of death.

I become a most diligent student, a zealous convert to the fact that *no*, cot bumpers are not safe and *yes*, do take flip-flops to the hospital to wear in the shower and *goodness*, whatever you do, don't forget to take Arnica for a week before delivery.

I judiciously debate the pros and cons of every form of pain relief and manage not to vomit or cry when we get to the bit where a shove from our instructor makes a rather battered plastic doll shoot out of an equally decrepit-looking plastic vagina.

Halfway through the class, we partake in refreshments of orange squash and bourbons. Snack time is signalled by a hand appearing round the door with a tray. Just a hand. Nothing more. We assume that it belongs to our teacher's other half, yet no one succeeds in spotting the rest of him – and a survey of many other acquaintances who have attended the same classes over the last decade and a half reveals that no one has ever managed a glimpse of anything beyond the elbow. But hey – at least this diverts focus from the photos of cone-headed infants that are handed round during the section on ventouse deliveries.

Towards the end of the evening, we practise our breathing and as we assume various 'pushing' positions everyone gets the giggles. Several of the husbands forget that they are the ones who are meant to be mopping brows, voicing encouragement and offering drinks with bendy straws, rather than actually giving birth themselves and they get rather too into the role play. There is a lot of hyperventilating and a lot more tittering before bed.

By now my bump is big and to squeeze behind the wheel of my car is no mean feat. As the weeks have passed, I've edged my seat further and further back to the point where I can't actually reach the pedals any more and have to take the bus instead.

There are recreational issues too. A girls' night out in a restaurant's fixed-seat booth ends in embarrassment as a combo of bump plus dessert means that by the end of the meal my stomach is wedged against the table and it takes two friends plus the manager to get me free.

Naturally, I am still managing to panic about the things that might go wrong, and because I dare not let myself think beyond a day at a time, my preparations for the birth are left quite late. With just a couple of weeks to go, a friend takes me on a shopping trip, piling my basket with little vests and sleepsuits and maternity pads. And cream for cracked and bleeding nipples. Which really does nothing for my nerves.

My husband and I head off to John Lewis and practise folding and unfolding prams, a skill which I appear to be incapable of grasping. The shop assistant demonstrates and with just a deft flick of the wrist my husband proves his own prowess in the art of perambulator erection.

And then it is my turn. I hold it up, I hold it down, I press, I twist, I sit on the floor and cry. My husband apologises to the crowd gathered around us and I am persuaded to have another go, but even then the result looks less like a pram than something a baby would need to be stuck to with industrial quantities of Sellotape in order to stay put. But we order one anyway, and a car seat too, though I insist that they are not delivered until the very last minute.

Friends tell me how they spent the last few weeks of their pregnancies knocking up casseroles and bakes to fill the freezer, but the very sight of fish, chicken, tomatoes and pasta still fills me with revulsion, so I compile a nifty folder of colour-coded pizza delivery menus instead.

There are more midwife checks, and I find myself wondering why the maternity unit has to be in the very farthest corner of the hospital, up several lifts and sets of stairs and along miles and miles of corridor. On a bad day it takes so long to trek the trek that you can see women wheeled into the labour ward with a bump and out again with a baby before you've even made it to the clinic. On one trip I've seen a woman who doesn't make it at all and gives up, lying down in the middle of the corridor shrieking with each contraction.

So when it is suggested that I can have my final checks at the GP surgery around the corner (12 stairs, no corridors) I gratefully accept.

Although I am still nervous and still panicking about the odd scare story that's managed to sneak past my husband's strict censorship, everything is good. He is busy at work, about to change jobs – while I am on maternity leave, supervising disruptive building work in the house (which appears to be de rigueur in the later stages of pregnancy) and being a lady who lunches (albeit not on pasta, chicken, fish …) for the first time in my life.

I roll round to the GP for my final check and casually mention that my shoulder's been giving me a bit of gip. Within seconds, we have switched from casual conversation to medical Monopoly mode: 'Go directly to hospital. Do not pass Go. Do not collect £200 … '

… And so here I am, in A&E, feeling right as rain (and therefore slightly fraudulent among my bleeding/puking/otherwise incapacitated compatriots), but clutching a note about a suspected pulmonary embolism. Due to having lost editorial control of the baby book, I have skipped the section on possible complications in favour of the bit about perineal massage, so I do not realise that my symptoms are potentially deadly and must always be investigated.

I am whisked into a cubicle and examined within minutes. I am aware that shoulder pain in early pregnancy can mean an ectopic, but eight and a half months in, with a stomach the size of a Pacific island, I figure that it's unlikely to be the problem on this occasion.

Blissfully unaware of the magnitude of this unfolding drama, I have brought nothing with me: no magazine, no phone charger, no change of clothes. So when I am admitted, it comes as a bit of a shock.

I have one bar left on my phone, just enough to call my husband who abandons his own leaving party to rescue his damsel in distress. I am on a general ward, far from the maternity unit and all alone in a side room that provides privacy and a shower, but no screening from the sounds of vomiting coming from the other side of the door.

The doctors liaise with the obstetrician and fill me in on the course of action: an overnight stay with various checks, an ultrasound of my limbs (a bilateral leg Doppler assessment, to those in the know) and a special scan that uses a radioactive substance to show how well oxygen and blood are flowing to all areas of my lungs.

I am uncharacteristically calm until I hear the word 'radioactive', then everything else becomes a blur as I panic about what will happen to the baby. But I am assured that the risks of the scan are outweighed by the risks of an embolism, and come the next morning I manage to hold my nerve as they inject me with the toxic fluid (although the radiologist does not actually respond when I ask him, 'How long until I start to glow?').

The scan itself is a pretty painless procedure and, thankfully, all is well, so I am wheeled down to a bed in the maternity unit while they work out what to do with me next.

But there is a problem. The curtains are hastily drawn around me and a midwife cautiously sticks her head in from the corridor to say that the radiation effectively means I am contaminated for the next 24 hours, and that during this time I must not have any contact at all with small children ... or pregnant women. I cannot stay on the ward.

'But *I* am a pregnant woman,' I shriek. 'How am I supposed to avoid having any contact with myself?'

Fortunately, I am saved – once again – by my consultant whose practical good sense sees me waddling home to rest, eat grapes and await the big day.

CHAPTER 2

HAPPY BIRTH-DAY

I have been booked in for a C-section, though I don't think that anyone who has ever set foot in this hospital would care to level the accusation that I am too posh to push. The Portland it ain't – and celebrities, en-suite facilities and celebration champagne dinners belong firmly in another world.

For years, I have watched friends agonise over birth plans, which have ranged from the lyrical (' … candles, soft music, aromatic spices and my husband gently stroking my forehead' – she ended up with an emergency section) to the prosaic ('Just give me an epidural and have done with'). Some eulogise about being at one with nature, some swear by HypnoBirthing, others get hooked on gas and air.

The options are endless – so perhaps it is good fortune that any decisions that I might have to make myself have been taken away from me on gynaecological grounds (a combination of my long-ago op and the fact that all that panting and pushing would apparently mean an increased risk of uterine rupture – gulp).

Knowing a section is the only safe and sensible option makes it easy for me to accept. (Especially when I hear friends' horror stories about rubber rings and infections and realise that post-birth stitches may be rather like small children – better to keep them where you can see them.) But given that older mums are far more likely to end up under the knife than their younger counterparts means that other friends have felt railroaded down this path.

A doctor friend explains that this is down to 'a combination of complications and/or the acceptance that as this may be the older mum's only pregnancy, there is a desire to try and ensure a good outcome'. Fine by me, though some chums still feel cheated out of the opportunity to try for a natural birth.

A 43-year-old of my acquaintance – let's call her Sarah (largely because that is her name) – recounts that through-out her pregnancy she was made to feel like a fossil.

'When I said I wanted to go for a regular birth they just kept telling me about all the problems I might come up against simply because I was in my 40s. It's really not what you want to hear when you're the size of a house and up to your armpits in hormones and haemorrhoids.'

There is little wonder that I feel a sense of relief as I bypass the labour ward for the operating theatre and, before I know it, am lying on a stainless-steel table, numb from the neck down, while a load of people in masks and rubber gloves appear to be removing my internal organs one by one. I hear shouts of, 'That's the bowel,' and, 'Here's the bladder,' as they dig towards my womb in a blaze of bright lights, accompanied by an unnerving soundtrack of suction, sploshing and strains of 'Drive' by The Cars – a song I have never liked.

And suddenly, a deafening yell as an angry, red, wrinkled infant makes sure its first task on earth is to protest about its eviction from my uterus.

It's a girl.

'She's a redhead,' says the surgeon, which is odd, given that my daughter has a full head of black hair.*

'You've given birth to your father,' says my husband, who is able to spot the family resemblance in an instant.

---

* ... which later falls out and grows back blonde (or at least mouse).

I'm still strapped to the table while some terribly nice medics play cat's cradle with my innards then try to put them all back where they belong. I try not to think about the time I took our broken radio apart, then found, when I'd screwed the front back on, that I had several parts left over.

I would like to say that I gaze lovingly upon my newborn daughter – but as she has been cleaned up, brought over and placed just beneath my chin, all I can actually see is a flailing red fist. Still, as first cuddles go, it feels pretty good.

Our new little family is wheeled/carried/pointed towards the recovery room where we are encouraged to bond.

I have had visions of these precious moments, picturing myself with beatific smile, bathed in a haze of golden light as I cradle my infant to my breast. The fact that I am morphined up to the eyeballs detracts from the reality, which is less golden haze, more fluorescent strip lighting. But no amount of drugs can diminish the sensation of the baby finding the nipple and latching on.

'Ooh – ferocious suck that one,' says a passing theatre nurse. But by this time I have entered a parallel universe, one in which it seems I have been captured by a bunch of sadists who have clamped my nipples into a vice and are now screwing its metal jaws tighter and tighter. And no one can hear me scream.

But back on planet Earth, the baby falls asleep and I can relax as I hold her warmth against me and everything is right with the world.

As evening draws on, my husband is sent home and the baby and I dispatched to the ward and settled into a curtained cubicle the size of a small dining table. There is a bed for me, a plastic goldfish bowl for the baby and a chair just big enough for a very thin visitor.

Although it is night, the ward is busy, noisy. I haven't eaten for 24 hours and the nurse disappears to see what's on offer. She returns with bread, jam and an apology – the toaster is broken and that's it until morning. Am too hungry to mind that the bread has not yet defrosted.

The propinquity of the other mothers is unnerving. We are packed so close together that if we drew back the curtains we would be able to count each other's stitches without leaving our beds.

Until the early hours I have no choice but to listen to the phone conversation of my neighbour, as she and her partner try to decide which member of the England football team to name their newborn son after. They finally settle on Rio – a definite improvement on the triple-barrelled Ashley-Wayne-Jermain, which is being mooted at one point.

The baby cries, and as I am shackled to the bed by a catheter, the nurse picks her up and brings her to me. She curls her tiny fingers around mine and for the rest of the night this is how we remain, she sleeping peacefully (and lulling me into a false sense of security) and me too frightened to breathe lest she loosen her grip and end this enchantment.

As dawn breaks, however, reality bites.

Over the course of my pregnancy, I have seen the very best of the NHS. My age has afforded me consultant-led care throughout. And while I may have worried myself into several sleepless nights over the statistics and scare stories surrounding older mums, my fears have always been gently allayed and my questions answered with endless patience.

Now, it seems, that cosseted existence is well and truly over.

The morphine wears off and the curtains are drawn back to reveal a long, almost endless line of beds in a crumbling ward that, even in its day, would have had

Florence Nightingale begging for a visit from Laurence Llewelyn-Bowen, MDF and all. I cannot move, still constrained by tubes and pouches and the fact that my legs seem to have run out of battery.

But it could be worse: three beds along, another mother is held captive for real – handcuffed to a prison officer who sits impassively as her charge struggles to manoeuvre her new baby to her breast with her one free arm. (The proximity of the hospital to the local jail means a steady stream of police officers passes back and forth throughout my stay – something I'm not quite sure what to make of, there not being a chapter in Gina Ford that even touches on post-partum prisoners.)

Other than that, it is not clear how this long ward is divided, although it would appear that there's a special Caesarean section for those of us who have had Caesarean sections. And I am positioned in its midst.

The woman to my left, who was sliced open right after me, leaps out of bed with the agility of an Olympic hurdler, runs around the room and says, 'Great – can I go home now please?'

And then it is my turn. Out comes the catheter and, 'Up you get,' says the nurse, dispatching me to the bathroom 75 miles away at the far end of the ward. But I have been so focused on the birth, on seeing the baby for myself and dispelling all my fears, that I haven't really considered what happens next.

Half an hour later, I still haven't managed to get both my legs off the bed and am wondering if I have somehow slept away a few decades without noticing and woken as a 90-year-old.

Slowly, slowly, one foot to the ground until, after considerable effort, both feet are on the floor. I shuffle them into my slippers and use the bedside table to try to lever myself into an upright position, not realising that it is on castors and thus shunting the baby into the corridor before landing in an undignified heap in the chair.

Finally, I am standing. Then it's just a matter of putting one foot in front of the other and setting out on my epic journey. By this time, I do not care that I am wearing only a hospital gown that is fastened at the back with just a couple of loose ties, and therefore largely open to anyone positioned at my rear; baring my disposable knickers to the world is the least of my worries. I am far more concerned with clutching the folds of my stomach to my chest, ensuring that my entrails do not fall out en route, for it feels like this is exactly what they are trying to do.

Twenty minutes later, I arrive at the bathroom to discover it is occupied. I would sit on the floor and weep, but the pain will not allow me to sink that far. Instead I wait my turn before collapsing on to the lavatory.

By the time I emerge, husbands, boyfriends and partners have been granted admission to the ward, so twice as many people get to see my outsize paper pants on the homeward shuffle.

I puzzle over how my neighbour is ready to run a marathon while I can barely make it back to bed. I blame my age, reassuring myself that she's young enough to be my daughter. Yet I can cling to this consolation only briefly: acquaintance through a gap in the curtains reveals that we are, in fact, contemporaries, geriatric mothers both.

In awe (or possibly shame), I furtively text friends who have also gone under the knife as over 40s to see if it really is just me. The odd one shares my pain: 'I dropped my soap on the way back from the shower and when another woman picked it up I thanked her and explained I'd just had a Caesarean. "Me too," she said, skipping jauntily down the ward without so much as a wince, leaving me thinking ah – that must be the difference that 20 years makes.'

However, the majority assure me that recovery is a breeze, and so I stagger back round the curtain, camp on the end of my new friend's bed and demand she let me in on the secret of eternal youth … I am still taking notes on exercise regimes, hair straighteners and the liberal use of Touche Eclat when my husband appears.

Back in bed, I cradle my daughter and we try out names. The only one we managed to agree on before the birth – Jacob – doesn't really cut it. We run through the list of also-rans, the ones we never quite saw eye to eye on,* and discover that my favourite – the one he had sworn against from the start – fits her like a glove. We try it with our surname, saying it over and over again in wonder as this little ball of Babygro and fluff suddenly becomes a person in her own right.

The baby demands food and I attempt to oblige. For more than a decade, I have watched friends suckle their young, nourishing their newborns tenderly at the breast, making the whole process look like a piece of cake.

Apparently, the cake is now stale. Or perhaps I should have been watching more closely, taking notes for future reference rather than making cups of tea, because

---

* This is perhaps an understatement. The neighbours may be able to verify that there were, indeed, some fairly heated differences of opinion. I blame the hormones and the fact that my husband does not always share my impeccable taste.

whichever way I try, it doesn't seem to be working. I hold her sideways, facing up, facing down. I try cushions for support, cushions for comfort – and cushions to bite down on when the pain gets too much. By now, my weeping is louder than the child's.

My husband suggests it may be baby blues and is so surprisingly forgiving when I throw my not-insubstantial copy of Penelope Leach at him that I blub some more.

The baby gets hungrier and hungrier, protesting loudly in an attempt to get her parents to rectify the situation. But we do not realise that although she is sucking for hours she is still not getting her fill. The hospital staff simply dismiss her as a 'hungry baby' and suggest I try to feed some more. But by this time I feel as though I have been taken over by my bruised and bloodied breasts and simply want to curl up in my G Cup and sleep away the pain.

I am also spending an inordinate amount of time trying to work out which way is up with the teeny, tiny nappies and how to change them without getting poo on the bed. A passing nurse seems surprised by my ineptitude, perhaps assuming from my age that I've done it all before. To be fair, I am also surprised at my ineptitude, given that over the last 15 years I have burped, cradled and comforted dozens of infants belonging to friends and family. Then I remember that at the merest hint of faecal imminence I've handed over said babies, cut and run. This, presumably, is payback time.

But actually, I realise that it's oh so true what they say: when it's your own it is very, very different. And I know no new mother – be she 18, 48 or anywhere in between – who has not spent these first few days slightly daunted and dazed by the responsibility, the reality.

With the unnerving immediacy of the other mothers, it is impossible not to eavesdrop on the conversations going on around me. The woman opposite is telling every-one with great pride that her boyfriend invented the name for their new bairn. And to be fair, she speaks the truth – certainly I never spotted 'Porschesky' (as in 'Por-shu. Sky') in any of the numerous naming books that I turned to for ideas. Two beds down has plumped for Ferrari. In fact, by the end of the day, it appears that my daughter is the only newborn on the ward not named after a footballer, a car or a booze-induced whim. In order that she should not feel left out, I suggest to my husband that we switch to Cantona-Cabriolet, but it is too late – my mum is striding towards us and there is no time for further discussion.

Although she is already a grandmother twice over, my mother is radiating pride and excitement to such an extent that she is glowing in a way that is strangely reminiscent of the Ready Brek kid. She is the first in a long line of cooing relatives eager to acquaint themselves with our child, and to offer counsel to her novice mother.

'Ooh, you'll need a few more cardigans than that,' says one, despite the fact that the temperature of the ward would make the Caribbean seem chilly. 'A nice jolly cot bumper's what you want,' says another. And a third chips in with, 'She'll sleep so much better on her tummy.'

I know from friends of all ages that new mothers are swamped with advice and instruction from their elders before the placenta's even been pushed out. But it is becoming clear that 40-odd years is a long time in childbirth. Times have changed and with them the doctrines of the NCT which I, as a new and zealous convert, believe I must obey unquestioningly at all times.

I try to explain politely that everything is different nowadays. That what worked when my husband and I were newborns is no longer the done thing several generations later. I wonder how many times one can say, 'It's just they tell you not to do it like that any more,' without destroying a beautiful relationship. But then the hormones kick in, I burst into tears and shout at everyone to leave me alone.

I am otherwise a dutiful patient, having been brought up old school to believe that rules are rules. 'No more than two visitors per bed at any time', reads a large notice at the entrance to the ward and I observe it with the caution of one who has grown up in the era of rulers across the knuckles.

The many younger mothers that surround me are, however, bolder, more carefree. One has so many people perched on the end of her bed that I am surprised that it doesn't capsize, spilling her dozens of relatives to the slightly sticky floor. Another is clearly flouting the no-kids rule, permitting only the newborn's siblings on the ward. She can't be more than 20, yet crowding into her cubicle is an assortment of youngsters, lined up in height order in a way that is uncannily reminiscent of that bit in *The Sound of Music* where Fräulein Maria first meets the von Trapp brood – only here there are no 'Doe, a deer's or 'Auf wiedersehen, goodbye's, just the odd crisp packet wafting into the corridor and an argument over a Slinky (presumably one of their 'favourite things').

A very nice nurse arrives and offers to show us how to bathe the baby. It looks easy enough – indeed, how complicated can something be when it only involves one small child, a bowl of warm water and a bit of cotton wool?

Apparently very complicated indeed. It doesn't go well.

Given that my husband has done all this once before (and done it rather well judging by the pleasing result),

I have been harbouring high hopes that he will be in a position to steer me through the worst of my incompetence. But it would appear that 14 years is long enough for him to have forgotten absolutely everything, and so we are forced to flounder together while the teenager looks on bemused, wondering how she made it through her own infancy unscathed.

Day Three in the Big Mother House. Only *just* Day Three, given that is five past midnight, but time is becoming immaterial. Extended visiting hours are granted to the fathers (their presence being permitted 9am–9pm), but the 12 hours that the baby and I spend alone each night seem like a lifetime and I rack up a mobile phone bill that will decimate the family allowance for months to come.

The baby is yelling and the night staff aren't happy.

'Can't you keep her quiet?' scolds the nurse, as though my daughter is a lone child disturbing the precious peace in a first-class cabin, and not one of 20, simultaneously shaking the foundations of a crowded ward.

Everyone is awake in any case. Everyone, that is, bar the woman opposite who snores with such force that I half expect Norris McWhirter to rise from the dead and congratulate her on her inclusion in the *Guinness Book of Records*. As night wears on, the decibels increase and the rest of us internees become united in adversity, exhausted beyond belief.

Each hour in the ward passes 20 times more slowly than those in the outside world and I clock-watch, counting the moments, the seconds until my husband can come back.

My lovely neighbour has been granted early release for good behaviour. And so I console myself by scrolling again and again through the many texts of congratulation I've received, though I'm not entirely sure who the one reading, 'Buxom Blonde – any time. Call 0800 Busty' is from.

Eventually, it is morning proper, discernible only by the fact that the slightly scary night staff have been replaced by the distinctly jollier day staff in a Jekyll/Hyde-type switch.

Breakfast awaits tantalisingly (or as tantalisingly as white bread and foil-wrapped butter pats can) in the kitchen, which is blessedly closer than the loo, but still a 15-minute slog each way. I am becoming increasingly concerned about my immobility and disheartened by the number of women (of all ages) around me for whom the Caesarean scar seems no more bothersome than a paper cut, while I feel like the lone survivor of the Texas chain-saw massacre.

I ring my husband (again) and ask him to Google some tips for recovery and he duly arrives with a sheaf of papers dispensing helpful hints …

'Hold a pillow to your tummy while you are doing a poo … ' suggests one website, presupposing you can make it to the bathroom in the first place, let alone lug a load of bed linen with you.

'Eat plenty of fruit and veg to keep those stools soft,' suggests another. So far, I have eschewed what's been on offer from the trolley – which might have been fruit and veg, hard to tell – in favour of Mars bars. But in order to show willing, I ask my husband to bring me a chocolate orange next time he pops to the shop.

'Don't forget! Regular pelvic-floor exercises!' advises a self-help forum. I am dimly aware that I must still have a pelvic floor somewhere between the top of my support stockings and my now pendulous breasts – but locating it among the stitches and maternity pads proves tricky.

Apparently, I should be rubbing creams, lotions and potions into my scar to stop it itching, but not only is it still under wraps, I am also so pathetically squeamish that I am not actually able to even look at it for another eight months.

One excellent site suggests that I ' ... ask the staff or a visitor to bring you some peppermint water to soothe the pain of trapped wind, which often follows surgery'. Sound advice – though it is an achievement to get a jug of tap water around these parts, and I can only imagine what would happen should I proffer this request. I guess someone might just toss in a Polo, but only on a good day.

I am also recommended to nick a pair of my husband's boxer shorts to accommodate my wound, but this just makes me laugh – and as I have forgotten to hold a pillow to my stomach to allow for this spontaneous outburst, the pain then makes me cry.

Every article warns that my emotions will be all over the place. And they are right. Pain and sleep deprivation are a heady mix, and now the baby is actually here I have traded my pre-birth panics for worries about the constant media reports and scares surrounding mid-life motherhood.

One says that our children may be prone to diabetes. Another that older mums are more likely to develop acute psychosis after birth. Every hormonal blip substantiates my fears and my husband feeds me yet another Mars bar in the hope that the endorphins might avert a crisis.

I have not yet braved the shower and am still bathed in the detritus of birth and afterbirth. There are a number of suggestions that ablutions may be the way forward, so off I stagger, armed with advice from the midwife on how to remove the dressing.

Slowly, slowly the gown comes off and … nothing. I cannot for the life of me work out how to turn on the shower. Gown back on, shuffle to nurses' station, receive instructions and shuffle back to bathroom. Gown off again, shower now working, a gentle flannelling of all the necessaries, then discover dressing stuck on with Super-glue and that tearing at even a corner of it feels like a bikini wax times ten. Leave wound covered, replace gown and stagger back to bed.

We have a surprise visitor – a former colleague who's here for an appointment of her own and has heard my news on the grapevine. She has popped in to present the baby with her very first gift, a tea towel – the hospital shop not offering much in the way of variety and the choice being either that or a copy of *Heat*. (And actually the tea towel has come in very handy, thank you.)

It is our final night on the ward and I wonder whether you can become institutionalised within the space of just three and a half days. I sleep (briefly, while the snorer is in the lavatory), and dream that I am in a Victorian workhouse and there is no escape. The outside world has disappeared and I am Oliver Twist, although given what's on offer from the trolley, it is very unlikely that I will be saying, 'Please Sir, I want some more.'

Then finally, finally we are granted release. The baby is strapped into her car seat for the very first time, hidden under the fluffy jacket that is purportedly for newborns, but which looks as though it will fit until she's at least nine months old. We are heading home and slowly, oh so slowly, our new little family begins the long walk to freedom.

CHAPTER 3

0–3 MONTHS

We are home.

The baby has been installed in a borrowed bouncy chair on one side of our living room and I have been installed on the sofa on the other. We are eyeing each other suspiciously – she wondering whether I have a clue what to do with her (no) and me trying to work out what on earth the various squeaks and snuffles are supposed to mean.

It soon becomes clear that a rough translation would be 'action at both ends', so while her father deals with the lower quarters, I bare my breast and position my pillow, hoping that it's all going to work better now we're home.

Apparently not.

Each suck sends a thousand razor-sharp daggers slashing through my nipple, and an hour later, when I have begun to hallucinate from the pain, she seems no more satisfied than before.

I ban all visitors and try every which way, but nothing quite seems to work. Ensconced in solitary confinement, we experiment further with cushions of every shape and size to cradle the child. Pillows here, pillows there, pillows blooming everywhere, but none in a position that heralds any form of success.

Using one of my three lifelines, I phone a friend. (And another one. And another …) Some have found it easy as pie, others marginally less painful than having a pencil rammed into your eyeball. But almost all have got there in the end.

I persevere.

A (male) neighbour arrives late at night with a (freshly sterilised) nipple shield for me to try. But all this does – other than destroy the last shred of dignity I had been clinging on to – is add another dimension to my ineptitude, as the baby still doesn't seem to be connecting in the right way.

The community midwife turns up and says, 'Goodness me, that baby looks like she's been Tangoed. Stick her by the window to get some sun on her – although it may be worth you taking her down to A&E for a check up while you're about it.'

So we do. They tell us she is jaundiced and to make sure she gets plenty of fluids. And so off we go home again and Velcro her to my bosom, instructing her to suck for all she's worth.

It's late at night and we are about to settle her in the crib beside our bed when she begins to vomit blood. I do what any new mother pumped full of hormones and stitches would do – cry. My husband takes charge and soon we are speeding back towards the hospital.

The baby looks very tiny there on the great big bed, so I cry a bit more and then a very nice doctor tells us that she is now severely jaundiced and needs to be admitted. But there are no beds, so we will have to be taken to another hospital up the road.

At three in the morning, we are swooping down hills that I had never thought of as swoopable (their being generally gridlocked during waking hours) and soon we are seeing yet more doctors and giving the baby a bottle to try and rehydrate her. She consumes it with gusto, then falls fast asleep as we watch the dawn break over London from the window of our room and take it in turns to try and snatch a few minutes' kip on the camp bed in the corner.

In the morning a breastfeeding counsellor arrives and spots right away that there is a problem. It does feel slightly odd to be making conversation with a complete stranger who is holding my (naked) left breast with one hand and poking my nipple in odd directions with the other, but at least she knows her stuff and can offer a diagnosis for the difficulties we have faced. It turns out that the baby has a tongue tie, which means it is impossible for her to latch on properly, so while she may well be sucking for Queen and Country, she's getting almost nothing in return. Except a lot of blood from me.

The medics fill her with formula instead and book her in for a corrective op. Meanwhile, the counsellor returns, wheeling a large and industrial-looking piece of machinery. She sticks suction cups over both my breasts and cranks up the power. For the next half hour, I am distracted from any aches and pains by the slightly unnerving sight of my nipples shooting up and down the plastic tubing. (Who knew they could stretch that far, eh? The things you never learn in biology …)

Meanwhile, throughout this entire episode, I am still at the mercy of my stiff, sore Caesarean wound. A friend has lent me a book on recovery from the procedure, but I haven't had time to open it, let alone take on board any tips it may offer to ease my discomfort. Though I am pretty sure that racing around hospitals in the dead of night and surviving on vending-machine snacks is not top of the list of 'must do's in terms of healing and regaining one's flexibility.

(Actually, now I think about it, perhaps I should write to the publishers to advise that any future editions should include a section on vending-machine posture: trust me – it's extremely tricky to bend down as far as the retrieval slot and make it back up again without dropping your Mars bar, which, in turn, simply throws up an entirely new set of issues.)

It is perhaps not surprising that by the time we make it home we are all a little battle-scarred and bewildered.

The days pass, and we are slowly settling into a routine. It has finally started to sink in that I am now a 'mum'. It's been a long time coming and I like the sound of the word immensely. However, the gloss is tarnished slightly by the community midwife's insistence that as I am the wrong side of 40, I must be described at every opportunity as an 'older mother'. I am, by now, only too aware of my advanced years, but I do not find this label flattering and do my best to come up with an alternative.

For 'old' perhaps 'antique'? After all, antiques are also on the aged side, yet they are both valued and cherished. I like to think that I too am valued and cherished, so does that make me an 'antique mother'? But on second thoughts, I decide that I'm not sure that this appellation does much for my self-esteem either.

My husband helpfully comes up with some ideas of his own. Though as he peruses the thesaurus throwing out synonyms such as 'decrepit' and 'dilapidated', I point out that 'divorce' also begins with a 'd', so perhaps that's as far as his trawl through the alphabet should go.

My morale is actually in need of a bit of TLC, as it happens. I have had nine months to forget the fact that there were a lot of baggy and saggy bits even before I embarked upon my gestational journey – and now I am beginning to realise that it's going to be an uphill battle to get rid of them, particularly given the amount of baby bulge that also seems to have stuck around.

It is not in the least bit helpful that the other members of my antenatal group – all many years my junior – seem to have pinged back into their size 10 jeans within 30 seconds of giving birth. I have not pinged for at least a decade, and it feels like it will take a miracle (or at least major surgical intervention) to get me out of my maternity wear and into anything with a zip.

I seek solace from the other aged mums who've been there too. 'It's your metabolism,' says one sagely. 'It slows down dramatically when you reach the big 4–0 you know.' 'Yes, definitely an age thing,' agrees another. 'Middle-aged spread meets motherhood? Way too much for a mere mortal to deal with. Go elasticated. That's my motto.' And, 'My skin's not so supple any more,' confesses a third. 'My baps are now baguettes. Mind you, I tell my new friends that I lost my figure since having my baby. No one need know I didn't have one to start with.'

The health visitor tells me that in one's teenage years and 20s one's muscles can just snap back into shape after having a baby – but once you hit your late 30s or 40s you're essentially buggered; I can see she's right – and that all those clichés of boobs and stomachs heading south are sadly true.

My friend Deb mournfully agrees: 'My pelvic floor needs retiling and my stomach will never again be a washboard substitute – though, on the bright side, it may come in useful as a trampoline.'

Ah well, at least I'm not alone … I feel greatly comforted until I meet up for coffee with my new mate from the maternity ward. I leave the house feeling fabulous. There is no puke on my stretchy trousers and I have even brushed my hair. Quite the glamour girl. I am mentally congratulating myself on progress made when the door of the café opens and a figure glides towards me straight from the pages of *Harper's Bazaar*. Glossy, sleek and svelte – oh so svelte.

When I choke out a few words of admiration she says, 'Well, everyone thinks keeping in shape is so much harder as you get older, but really, with a bit of motivation, it's not that bad at all. Mind you, it did take me a whole month this time round, so maybe my age is against me after all … '

I rearrange my child to cover my bulging midriff and order a large piece of chocolate cake as consolation.

The baby has now had her tongue-tie op, which mainly involved sitting around in a very warm room with lots of other infants and parents and then trooping en masse through the bowels of the hospital to the operating theatre where the small fry were snipped, one by one, as we grown-ups sat outside and tried to put a brave face on it. ('They don't even bleed most of the time,' said the nurse in charge, which seemed to be true until it came to our turn and I cuddled the baby to my chest for comfort, whereupon she dripped bright red blood all over my favourite T-shirt.)

We have had to bottle feed in the interim, but I am attempting to keep my milk supply going by becoming the third of my circle of friends to borrow my best mate's breast pump – trying not to think of all the other nipples that have been forced into submission by this groaning mechanical beast.

Yet I now fully understand the phrase 'blood out of a stone' and become truly dispirited at the minuscule amount of milk that ends up in the bottle.

I dream that I am being taunted by my box of breast pads. 'You'll never need us,' they cry savagely, as I stuff whole handfuls of the things down my nursing bra in a bid simultaneously to silence them and to remove them from my eye line.

A friend (an earth mother who puts me to shame with her cloth nappies, homemade wet wipes and freezer full of organic placenta fritters) suggests I try expressing milk by hand. She emails me a diagram of a woman squeezing her nipple into a glass together with a set of comprehensive instructions on how to place my fingers around my areola and massage, pull and push in assorted directions and at varying speeds to get my milk ducts flowing. She has, however, forgotten that I have the co-ordination of a carthorse trying to ballet dance in clogs: after an hour's worth of pushing, pulling and trying to match the postures in the picture, I have succeeded only in mashing my mammaries until they hurt too much to touch – and there's not so much as a drop to show for my troubles.

I go to a breastfeeding clinic, where an assortment of new mothers of all ages sit around weeping over their incompetence and placing their errant breasts and babies (quite literally) in the hands of the counsellors in charge. At least I am momentarily sidetracked from my own shortcomings by the rantings of a mother who is refusing to accept the advice that she needs to think about cutting back on the boob because her child is due to start school (and apparently it's not the done thing to breastfeed through the railings). It takes me every ounce of self-control not to shout out, 'Bitty' and run.

As instructed, I follow the clinic's diet sheet (Mars bars? What's not to like?) and their advice to pump at regular intervals, including at least one session between midnight and 6am. I pump alone, to the accompaniment of endless episodes of Sky-Plussed *Coronation Street*, and to the exclusion of sleep and social life, yet at the end of each day I am lucky to have accumulated enough for one measly feed and formula has to do the rest.

When I accidentally drop a bottle of the priceless nectar all over the floor, thus negating a total of two hours at the milking machine and precious time I could have spent sleeping, it is truly the final straw.

My oldest friend Jo does her best to offer some words of comfort, attributing my difficulties not to my lack of lactation but to post-traumatic stress syndrome as a result of an unfortunate breast-related incident involving her pet rabbit Harvey.

To spare myself unnecessary angst and to minimise the flashbacks, I shall not go into too much detail, but suffice to say that I was wearing a (tight-fitting) green sweater, the day was cold and the bunny took my nipple for a tempting new variety of salad leaf. One minute he was happily (and harmlessly) lolloping across the floor, the next his teeth were firmly clamped around my bosom.

I would like to say that both my lifelong friend and my husband were sympathetic to the fact that I almost lost my breast to a lop-eared dwarf, but alas this would be a lie and it pains me to report that they were, in fact, laughing too much to be of any assistance whatsoever.

Little wonder then that at the six-week check the doctor pronounces the baby to be thriving, then takes one look at the stress-induced hives all over my chest and tells me that in this case bottle is best.

I am devastated – particularly when well-meaning friends tell me how they managed to struggle on even when their nipples fell off and their boobs got infected and grew to the size of Sardinia and other such horrors. But I am also not prepared to let the baby starve, and so formula it is – even if it means I now don't get to watch *Corrie* for weeks due to my no-TV-with-baby-in-the-room rule.

To cheer me up, my husband has planned a trip up North so we can see my family and show off the child. Relatives and friends all gather from afar and the baby does her bit by ensuring that her infant acne and cradle cap are at their peak for the visit. Alas, the child is too young for concealer, and it is unseasonably warm, which means a hat to cover the offending flakes is also out – so all in all, she's not looking her best.

This is a shame as my mother spends most of our trip with the baby out in the open, for all the neighbours to see, proudly wheeling her up and down the road in my old pram – an enormous wooden contraption as old as the hills and so large that it can be seen from space.

Fortunately, I am too busy revelling in a succession of home-cooked meals to care about anything else. And my husband, whose allergy to the family pet has left him cowering behind a large box of tissues and a stack of anti-histamines, is in no position to demur.

We hold court on a sunny Sunday afternoon and a succession of aged ladies, who raised their own children in the days before centimetres had even been invented, take it in turns to tell us exactly how to bring up baby ...

'You should mix a load of baby rice into her bottle,' says an ancient aunt. 'That'll get her sleeping through.' 'Shall I give her just a teeny weeny bit of chocolate from my finger?' asks another as I run screaming from the room in order to remove my child from harm's way.

When we return, we are taken aside by an old family friend who has apparently kept her copy of Dr Benjamin Spock's *The Common Sense Book of Baby and Child Care* welded to her bosom since 1958 (either that or she desperately needs a better bra). 'I wanted to tell you,' she begins, 'that it is very important that the baby is nice and toasty at all times, but especially at night. A lovely fluffy cap at bedtime ... '

Personally, I think that it is very important that I stand on the sofa right this minute and shout very loudly that this is actually the 21st century and that everything has changed.

It is no longer in vogue to dangle a newborn over a potty as an encouragement. (And yes – this really happened; bear witness to one grainy black and white photograph, circa 1965, in which yours truly, aged one week and one day, is being suspended in just such a fashion. Total waste of time by the way – I was still wetting my knickers by the time I went to nursery.)

Nor is it all the rage to feed toddlers buttered bread sprinkled with sugar. Not that my mum ever did, I should add before she disowns me – although I do recall looking on with envy as other parents bespeckled their children's bread with gay abandon, as was the fashion of the day.

Nowadays, we do not lay carrycots across the back seat of the car without restraint as 'everyone did when you were that age', according to my parents and everyone else I meet of their generation. Small boys are not forced to wear short, short trousers and knee socks, even in the dead of winter (but oh – how I get to chuckle at the photos of my brother and his goosebumps, so perhaps that wasn't all bad after all). And the food office no longer makes you dose your baby on cod liver oil and rose hip syrup.

I want to shout that it is a very long time since I was a nipper, even longer since most of the assembled throng has been anywhere near to childbearing age and, once again, *we do it all differently these days, thank you very much* ... But my husband restrains me with a large plate of florentines, so instead I end up having to smile politely and say, 'More tea?' or 'Another slice of cake?' seething inwardly all the while, and thus dramatically increasing my chances of an ulcer.

I guess it does not help that my hormones are still in overdrive. Every day I seem to shed enough hairs to stuff a small cushion; then there are the hot flushes to boot. Once again, I spend every spare minute on the Internet trying to work out whether the cause is new motherhood … or menopause.

Could it really be The Change? I scroll through the symptoms …

- Menstrual irregularity? Check.
- Sleep disturbance? I have a newborn. Of course my sleep is bloody disturbed (though the website doesn't clarify whether this actually counts …).
- Mood changes? Judging by the fact that if my husband has anything even remotely controversial to ask me he now stands outside in the garden and telephones through his request, I would say yes, check.
- Joint pains? My knees have been shot since halfway through my pregnancy. I've been blaming the baby … but could it be that Old Mother Middle Age should be taking the rap instead?

- Hot flushes? Thinning hair? Check, check.
- Weight gain? How am I supposed to tell under all these layers of baby belly?

I am not yet ready to renounce my youth. Nor am I ready to embrace crimplene and candlewick and buy a slow cooker. I want to read *Grazia*, not *Woman's Weekly*. I want to deny the fact that I think, Ooh, how practical, when I see magazine advertisements for slip-on shoes ...

I ring the doctor.

Apparently, it is a false alarm and everything is fine. It seems that these are all perfectly normal occurrences in women who have just given birth. But then owing to the iron curtain being drawn around all my baby manuals, I guess there is no way I would have known that.

And so I get on with being a mummy. By trial and error and yet more phone calls to friends who've done this all before me, I start to find my feet. At long last, I get to grips with changing nappies and I learn to tell the difference between the baby's 'I need milk and I need it NOW' expression and the one that says, 'Can't you give a girl some privacy when she's trying to poo?'

Even better: I finally get to sit down and eat a whole meal all in one go and, as the summer sets in for real, I wheel my pram in the sunshine and rock and coo like a natural.

The baby is very well behaved, given her lineage; she sleeps when she is meant to and eats when she is meant to, which is lucky as it's just about the only way I can work out what I'm doing. Feeding and sleeping are at precise and regular intervals (and noted on paper for good measure), and in between the baby splits her time between cooing under the gaily coloured arch of the borrowed baby gym and vomiting over her parents. All this as I struggle to come to terms with night feeds and early mornings and gradually lose the plot.

'Shhh, shh, can't you see I am feeding the baby?' I snap at my husband when he wakes me one morning, only to discover that it is actually a pillow that I am cradling to my (empty) breast while whispering sweet nothings of encouragement.

A younger friend tries to comfort me by telling me it won't be long until I get my mojo back. But I find this confuses me all the more: as far as I am aware a Mojo is a small chewy sweet that comes in strawberry, orange and cola flavours and can be found between the white mice and foam shrimps in any self-respecting sweet shop's 'penny corner'. (More to the point, I've found them very hard to come by since I moved down South, where no one under 30 seems to have even heard of them. In desperation, I ring the manufacturers in Blackpool and ask if I can obtain a list of stockists closest to home, so hopefully all will be well that ends well.)

In the meantime, however, I find myself rocking and shh-shing the supermarket trolley to keep it asleep, when all it contains is a mango and an aubergine – the baby being safe at home with her dad.

For some reason that I cannot now remember we decide to swaddle the baby at night. Perhaps this is a throwback to our own babyhoods all those years ago, when it was very much the done thing. Or perhaps it is because it's what the nurses did in the hospital, wrapping her so deftly in her little cotton blanket that we figure why not?

But the answer to this question becomes immediately apparent – because we are absolutely and completely rubbish at it.

It's not so bad in the early evening when we do it with the light on before settling her down to sleep. But come the middle of the night, when we are fuzzy headed with sleep and can't see what we're doing, it's another story altogether.

Because she is sleeping in our room it becomes an impossible challenge to reparcel the child efficiently while cursing quietly enough not to wake whoever gets to stay in bed on any given occasion. It's a bit like *The Krypton Factor* on mute – and we are the losers every time.

Sure, it may not be rocket science, but it seems to me that it's every bit as complicated. Fold, fold, tuck, tuck, fold … it's almost like origami, except in crocheted cotton. Indeed, I become rather adept at making boats and hats and those nifty little fortune-tellers out of blanket – but never at keeping the baby snug and secure overnight.

And so it is that around four o'clock each morning we are woken by a low growl as the baby does her Harry Houdini act, followed by a triumphant gurgle as she waves her fists in the air as if to say, 'Free again! You two really don't know what you are doing, do you?'

We buy a Grobag.

Everyone tells me how lucky I am that (despite her parents) the baby has settled into the way of things quickly, up only when it's time for a routine refuelling. All the same, I am discovering that night feeds at 40 are no joke.

Truth be told, I have never been one for an all-nighter, and even in my younger days would generally opt for cosy bed and book over dancing till dawn. So as a confirmed dormouse rather than a night owl, it's difficult to tell how much – if any – of my all-consuming exhaustion is down to my age. Perhaps in my 20s, even early 30s, I might have been slightly less of a disaster without my eight hours' sleep? But alas, I will never know.

All I can tell you is that now, like an alcoholic smuggling a bottle of sherry in her handbag, I become obsessed with trying to grab a furtive 40 winks at any opportunity, appropriate or not.

At a family lunch, for example, I offer to take everyone's jackets upstairs – and my husband finds me half an hour later snoring gently under a pile of coats. I am surprised by how unimpressed the rest of the gathering is; personally I consider it rather resourceful to make the most of every chance I get.

In desperation, I offer to sell my soul for just half an hour's kip – but it seems that souls are 10 a penny these days for I don't even get a sniff of an offer.

Although I am a mid-life mum, the funny thing is that it does not seem to be the tiredness that is making me feel my age. Nor even the grey hairs, which now seem to be appearing with unnerving regularity, despite my regular trips to the hairdresser to slather them with copious amounts of dark brown gloop.

Nope – it's music that gets me. Every time.

None of my new friends have even heard of half the people in my record collection. Come to that, half of them have never even heard of *records*, having been born into an age where CDs are the norm and vinyl is something you are only likely to find on the kitchen floor.

They did not spend their youth slow dancing to 10cc and Fern Kinney, nor did they march around primary school singing, 'I am a cider drinker' (in a very poor West Country accent) – which, now I think about it, was fairly inappropriate on a number of levels, so perhaps it is best to move on.

I quiz my mum chum Amelia (31, no grey hairs, heart-stoppingly hip). 'Come on, you must have heard of *some* of these? Norman Greenbaum? Styx? Anita Ward? Kelly Marie? You must have heard of Kelly Marie? She did for flying suits what Delia did for cranberries and liquid glycerine.'

'What are flying suits?'

I tell her that I am depressed that I am so obviously untrendy, to which she replies (after looking me up and down in assessment), 'At least you've got a cool kitchen. Oh – and by the way, no one says "trendy" any more.'

I spend the rest of the week brushing up on my urban slang in a bid to get down with the kids, but it must be said that I do get some slightly strange looks when I greet my husband publicly with: 'Boom boom buzzin' buff boy, you looking well chung, but that shirt is so bait it's howling.'

I find it funny to think that had I lived in Roman times at my age I would most likely be a great-grandmother – or dead – by now. But in the noughties things are oh so different. I may be closer (much closer) to qualifying for a Saga holiday than an 18–30s, but I am also a new mum in an age where that really isn't so out of the ordinary.

A doctor friend agrees that there is no doubt that the cultural norms are changing. Life expectancy is increasing and the population, by and large, is not only older, but more active than ever before (and actually yes, in my old life I do recall once interviewing a parachuting granny who was planning an assault on Everest …).

But (and why does there always have to be a but?), he adds that we can bungee jump off the Empire State Building or run marathons for all we're worth – however unless the average age of menopause rises (which it shows no sign of doing) it won't make the blindest bit of difference to our ovaries: 'All women are born with a fixed number of eggs and before they are even born and during childhood the numbers begin to decline.'

I look around at the many older mums I know and think how very lucky we are, not only to have eggs that have hung on in there, but also to exist in an era where we can be out and proud. Women giving birth in their late 30s and early 40s have never had it so good.

After talking to a cousin who gave birth at the age of 44 in the far-from-liberal mid-50s, I count my blessings all the more. 'I was mortified,' she says. 'I was made to feel so embarrassed about hanging nappies on my line at my time of life that I had to get my neighbour to pretend they were hers instead.'

And a family friend, who had her youngest in the early 1970s when she was 42 found that even then she became a figure of fun:

'Everyone thought it was hilarious that at my age I was going to have a newborn. Luckily my son never had a problem with it. In fact, at primary school, when the children were asked to write a story about their mothers, he wrote, "I am very proud of the fact that I have the oldest mum in the class." He's always said it is his claim to fame!'

Of course, I have listened to enough radio phone-ins to know that even in these (supposedly) enlightened times there will always be those who think that a woman's ovaries should be put out to pasture the minute she hits her 30s. And yes, I fully understand that if all your mates have done with the sprog popping by the time they're 25, you really are going to be the odd one out if you're busy hatching while their kids are going off to college or walking down the aisle.

But actually, given the fact that the *average* age of procreating in the UK is now nigh on 30, I haven't managed to work out why the soap-box brigade get quite so het up about it in any case.

It's a regular subject of discussion at our girls' nights out.

'For goodness sake – it's not like I'm some sixty-something who is giving birth to twins the same day her pension book arrives,' says Jenny (second baby at 42). 'It's so common these days. And hair dye blurs the age gap to a large extent in any case.'

And Claudia (40 – Italian) weighs in with the fact that in Italy one in every 20 babies is born to a mum in her 40s and it's totally accepted – so what's the big deal about it over here? 'I know I left it late – but is that really anyone else's business? I met one woman who got really stroppy and said it wasn't fair that I'd been able to have fun, date lots of men, stay thin and have a career and now I was going to get the reward of having kids as well. I'm not sure she needed to get quite so uptight about it – but yes, we are a lucky lot who have been able to have the best of both worlds ... '

I think of friends who have not been so lucky – who have not been able to beat the biological clock for a whole host of reasons – and I feel very very fortunate to have my gorgeous girl waiting for me at home.

Nonetheless, the baby seems determined to put my maternal commitment to the test and develops a propensity for projectile poo that would challenge even the most dewy-eyed of mothers.

For the most part, I am adept at averting disaster. Indeed, my hand–eye co-ordination improves no end, and I wonder whether this might qualify me for a wild-card entry for Wimbledon. But one day I take my eye off the ball, remove the nappy without thinking and splat ... my hands are full of the stuff. Copious amounts of foul-smelling goo also cover the changing table, the carpet, the curtains, my clothes, the baby's backside and the fan on the floor, which, thank the lord, is not switched on – though it has gone through every little section of the grille and is dripping off the blades on to the floor.

I dare not disappear to empty my armful in case the child falls off the table so I scream, loudly, until my husband appears.

'I see the shit hit the fan,' he says before collapsing with mirth. He is absolutely no help whatsoever.

It takes an entire hour to complete the poo removal; the fan is too far gone for any hope of recovery and is laid to rest in the wheelie bin.

Although we have eschewed the idea of a proper summer holiday, now seems like a good time to take a little break. We book a cottage in the Peak District and, having loaded up the car with all the essentials, we then realise there is no room left for the baby and have to start all over again.

The sun shines throughout our stay, although, truth be told, we seem to spend as much time loading the washing machine as we do admiring the scenery. And if we are not as tanned as we might have been it is because of the disproportionate amount of time we spend indoors trying to fix the portable blackout blind to the window of the bedroom in order to disguise the fact that, with it being summer, the sun is rising an awful lot earlier than it really needs to.

The portable blackout blind is truly a genius invention – although in the hands of incompetents such as ourselves it does lose a certain *je ne sais quoi*. No one else I ask seems to have the slightest bother in fitting it to windows of any size or persuading the suction cups to suck, but somehow, as soon as we get hold of it, it all becomes a little haphazard.

And then there's the two-windows-one-blackout-blind factor to contend with which requires the careful but copious use of black bin bags and Sellotape and ensures that the rest of one's holiday is spent in permanent darkness where day becomes night becomes day.

Aside from that though, a good time is had by all.

Some friends have bought us a mobile as a gift and now that we're back from our trip we affix it to the baby's crib to allow her to fall asleep to strains of Bach, Beethoven and Mozart in melodic bite-size chunks.

Each night, we carefully darken the room to differentiate night from day, put the baby to bed and press Play. For some reason (that I have yet to fathom), we decide that the music needs to run for at least an hour to enable the child to drift into deep sleep. And so, precisely 14 minutes and 30 seconds after we have left her, we must sprint back up the stairs, perform a combat-style wiggle across the floor in order to remain unseen and hit the button, just as the final bars are chiming, so as to start up another 15 minutes of soothing lullaby. This process must be repeated a minimum of three times.

And then one night we forget. And it makes precisely no difference whatsoever.

Fortunately, the baby's good nature continues to compensate for any inadequacies on her parents' part. She has now learned to smile and in my efforts to keep track of every nuance of her development I am snapping so much that any paparazzo would be proud. This is largely because I am keen to capture every moment I can for the family album, but partly also because I have discovered that Facebook (which I had hitherto believed to be a social networking website) actually turns out to be a competitive sport and it is imperative that I prove my child's leaps in progress on a daily basis.

While, unlike some, I am loath to chart my daughter's every bowel movement with a tweet, I do figure that if you're in for a penny, you might as well go in for a pound and sign myself up for a whole load of 'mummy' websites for good measure.

My husband is alarmed to return from work to discover that I'm so busy multi-tasking (juggling a forum on the merits of digestives v. Rich Tea with another on whether soft toys on grown-ups' beds are right or wrong (oh so wrong) and a chat room confab about restoring one's bosoms to their former prime) that I have forgotten to feed the baby.

Now that my Caesarean scar is pretty much healed and I have found my feet as much as I'm ever going to, I am keen to get out and about at every opportunity. To this end, the pram that we have bought is one that allows us to remove the carrycot thingy and clip the car seat on to the buggy frame for ease of passage between vehicle and outside world.

Of course, this sounds as though it is perfectly simple and straightforward. But, naturally, it is not. Even remotely.

Firstly – without the woman in the shop there to demonstrate or my husband there to do it for me – I need to work out how to unfold the chassis. You would think that this could be done without a degree in mechanical engineering, but apparently not. I realise that this is why the damned thing came with an instructive video, and curse myself for not making the time to watch it.

Secondly – the clips. There is one clip to go on the 'prong' thing on the right and, correspondingly, another to go on the 'prong' thing on the left. But is that left and right as you look at it or left and right if you are sitting in it? Trial and a lot of error (plus my husband explaining it to me again and again) have not equipped me with the answer to that particular question.

Thirdly – the car seat is heavy and swinging it on to said clips without a crane or a second pair of hands is an uphill battle for someone with a dodgy back and the dexterity of a clown in a straitjacket.

Fourthly – is not the point of said contraption to allow baby to snooze on in its car seat while you lug it round the supermarket/to a meeting/to watch you get your corns done (delete as applicable)? And yet the labour entailed in the process of its erection is guaranteed to ensure that said child is wide awake and screaming before you have even reached step three.

It is infinitely easier just to stay home.

However, the health visitor has told us that we must attend the baby clinic on a regular basis, and because my old-school obedience is still switched to full power, I duly mark out the dates in my diary then carve them in stone for good measure.

Consequently, as soon as the home visits have stopped I sally forth for our first weigh-in, soaking up the sunshine as I wheel my pram jauntily beneath blue skies for the mile and a quarter to the clinic, rejoicing in the fact I don't have to go near the bloody car seat.

My high spirits are short lived. For what the health visitor failed to mention is that buggies must be left outside.

There is obviously some sort of conspiracy afoot, for every other perambulator is neatly padlocked to the railings, whereas the last thing I have thought of packing in my oversized bag of baby essentials is any form of security device.

I sneak into the downstairs doctor's surgery only to be accosted by the receptionist asking how I have the audacity to bring my buggy over the threshold. Head hung low I meekly ask if there might be a place to buy locks in the vicinity.

And so it is back out into the heat of the day to search for the bicycle shop in question.

We walk up, we walk down, we walk all around, then up and down some more – but there is no sign of the store.

This is possibly because it closed down two years earlier.

Time is running out and I am drenched in sweat and starting to hyperventilate from stress. I try the hardware shop ('Sorry – there's been a run on them'; DEFINITELY a conspiracy). I try Argos. I try the florist (probably as much down to sunstroke as desperation).

With 15 minutes left until the clinic closes a helpful newsagent tells me of a bicycle shop he knows that is definitely open. But it is a mile and a quarter away – *at the end of my road*!

Just as I am about to sink to the pavement in a sticky mass of sweat and tears, there it is: a shop full of grilles and safes and spikes and … locks. I assume that it is a mirage, but when I push the door it feels solid enough and soon I have my bounty in my hands.

I make it back to the health centre, work out how to open then secure the lock, retrieve the baby and suitcase full of nappies and bottles, after which I have to fight my way through a posse of young, glamorous and not-in-the-least-bit-sweaty mums on their way out. We fall out of the lift and into the clinic just as it closes – but the health visitors are a kindly species and taking one look at me decide I am in need of assistance.

One whisks away the baby to give her a bottle. The other makes me a cup of tea, which she hands over with lots of soothing comments that I am too busy weeping to hear.

But all is well that ends well: the baby does get weighed and we do make it the mile and a quarter home, whereupon I email everyone in the area who is pregnant, may be pregnant or is even considering getting pregnant and urge them to buy a bicycle lock.

CHAPTER 4

3–6 MONTHS

Funny the things that stick in your mind. Nothing useful, of course.

These days, I appear to be incapable of remembering to pay the gas bill or pick up more nappies from Tesco. It slips my mind that Monkey is surface clean only and turns rabid when you put him in the washing machine. Squeeze him once he's been through the spin cycle and for weeks to come he'll foam white, soapy suds from the mouth.

Yes, these days I forget anything of any consequence – so why is it that I am able to recall in great detail the entire contents of my friend Joanne's wardrobe between 1976 and 1979 (including a much-envied and rather fetching purple dress and mustard leather belt combo)? I know the telephone number of the house we moved out of when I was seven (although not the one where we have lived for the last four years) and the lyrics to the album *Wombling Songs*, which was very big in Manchester in 1973 let me tell you.

I believe it was track three (side one) that proclaimed, 'Exercise is good for you, laziness is not'. And finding myself idly humming it about the house one summer day I decide that this might be a sign that it is time to impose this edict upon my daughter.

You can't start too young, so I'm told. Which is why the minute the four-month jabs are out of the way, my wee girl is being bundled into a swimming nappy for the commencement of a term of classes.

And the pool is a winner. She loves it. Possibly to drink more than to swim in, but no matter. She splashes. She squeals with delight. She slurps some more. In her eyes, every aspect of the class is a hit. Though as the youngest by far, she copes less well with the instructor's directives than some of the others.

'Hold on to the bar and use it to help you climb out,' he commands. Being unable to sit or stand – let alone climb – doesn't help her any. Not knowing what a bar is probably adds to the confusion (though she is seen giving it a cursory lick which I feel enters into the spirit, if nothing else).

Week Two, and as we parade towards the pool I overhear one of the other mothers confide, 'If my husband

knew I'd come here without waxing he would throw a fit.'
I count my blessings that my own dear spouse is simply
content that we make it through class without drowning
and that hair removal issues are way off the agenda.

Indeed, I never do get to grips with the whole
yummy-mummy-by-the-pool look that everyone else
seems to have perfected with such splendour. Nor do I
understand how, as winter comes ever closer with freezing winds swirling in from the Steppes, each and every
one of them sports a healthy golden glow when the best
I can manage is duck-egg blue with goosebumps. And
while they strut to the poolside with the poise of catwalk
models, I slink gracelessly behind, asking myself how a
woman who has given birth just two weeks ago (teeny
baby with nanny on poolside as proof) could have a
stomach as flat as any athlete, when four months on my
own midriff is more reminiscent of Bernard Manning.

Still, on the bright side, the lessons are a great
success, and the baby takes to aquatics like the prover-
bial duck to water.

As for me, I spend the entire term trying to work out
how the other mothers manage to shower, dress and
blow dry – yes, blow dry! – with their dried-and-dressed
offspring in tow. Try as I might, my daughter is always
slightly soggy for the homeward trek. And by Week

Three I have learned that abandoning any niceties (including my undies and socks) is the only way I can get us both out of there the same day.

Inclement weather puts paid to a second term, the thought of venturing anywhere without smalls being enough to forsake the booking fee forthwith. Instead, we master other sports over the winter – sitting, standing and stair climbing, to name a few.

However, the timing of this newfound activity is unfortunate: as my daughter's mobility increases, so mine decreases. The bad back, which has been threatening revolt for some time, now goes for an all-out strike – protest, perhaps, at being dragged through the stresses and strains of pregnancy at an age where most women are as likely to be thinking about osteoporosis as offspring.

As if to prove my point, the postman arrives with another bunch of direct mail. It would seem that gone are the days of speculative invitations to health spas and fashion shows – now they (whoever these anonymous marketeers may be) are trying to tempt me with offers of bone-density scans and half-price discounts on calcium supplements.

Though I hate to admit it – perhaps they know me better than I know myself. For lugging a larger-than-average baby around in a car seat proves to be the final straw, and out and about one morning I suddenly find myself crippled by a pain that has me sweating and weeping in equal measure.

Somehow, I make it back to where I've parked the car, but getting the baby back in is another matter altogether. The street is deserted and it has started to rain, so sprawling on the pavement and sobbing until a rescuer arrives is not really an option.

With superhuman effort, I manage to bundle us both into the back seat and finally the baby is strapped securely in place. Crying and cursing, I half crawl to the front door and lever myself into my seat.

We eventually make it home (at least as soon as the road works on the A1 allow), where help is at hand. My mother-in-law takes the baby and I haul myself over the threshold looking uncannily like a cowboy who's just taken the full force of an Indian's arrow – all bow-legged and staggering before the obligatory (yet dramatic) slump to the floor.

The recovery is tortuous, but with a baby to care for there is no choice but to grit my teeth and get on with it. A scan, an epidural, a pair of crutches and a lot of drugs see me through the worst, and I gratefully accept all offers of assistance.

I have a brief moment of inspiration as I think of Peter Pan (perhaps the codeine?) and recall that Nana, the dog, had carted her charges around in her teeth. But I soon discover that human crowns are no match for canine dentistry and ring my mum instead.

Before long, and thanks in large part to a steady intake of ibuprofen, we are back in the social whirl that is new motherhood.

Within weeks of the baby being let loose on other people's soft furnishings, I discover she has 'a reputation'.

Not, alas, for her sweet nature, her winning smile or even the hearty chuckle, which sounds uncannily like the expectorant hack of a 100-a-day smoker. No. While all concerned duly note these virtues, they are sadly superseded by her status as 'the vomit comet'.

As other mothers blithely pass their babies round and bounce them on their knees without so much as a muslin or pair of galoshes in sight, I can only look on with incredulity. My sociable little daughter (who, it appears, adheres firmly to the maxim, 'What goes down must come up') may be happy to be handed round any number of friends and family, but every cuddle comes with a warning and a waterproof.

I have already blown most of my maternity allowance on getting the sofa steam cleaned and I have learned the hard way that an excellent exercise for post-Caesarean recovery is getting down on all fours to clean white puddles off friends' carpets, while apologising profusely. I find myself regularly pretending to drop my keys in restaurants so I can mop the floor without drawing attention to the curdling deposit at my feet.

The trouble is getting up again afterwards – although perhaps this is simply another reminder that at my age my time would be better spent with me reclining gracefully on a chaise longue or taking gentle strolls by the river.

Thanks to my nauseous nipper, my wardrobe has had a revamp. Anything marked 'Dry Clean Only' has been taken to the charity shop and I've come to regret the number of black tops that seemed, at the time, an essential requirement of my former media lifestyle.

Our record so far is four T-shirts (each) within 15 minutes, and while we have had to order a new washing machine (the old one expired from exhaustion), I am still bemused by the fact that nowadays I pack more clothes to pop out for a quick coffee than I used to for a week's holiday in Spain. I'm thinking of getting her sponsored by Fairy non-bio …

In terms of practicalities, I am learning many lessons:

- Do not visit anyone with carpets.
- Choose wellingtons over open-toed sandals.
- And Febreze Summer Splash truly does eliminate odours and freshens with a fruity summer scent.

In fact, all in all, I think I cope pretty well – though there is a moment of upset at an NCT reunion when our host refuses to have the baby photos taken on her new sofa if my malodorous minx is included in the line-up. The child responds to the insult by throwing up on the Persian rug instead – so I figure that makes us quits.

Although endless apologies and generous use of wet wipes make amends on this occasion, I am discovering that there are other times when my new chums and I do not see eye to eye.

Whether our disagreements boil down to nature or nurture I cannot say, though I do suspect that it's that (semi-) generational thing rearing its slightly greying head once again.

Allow me to offer an example.

Long ago, in the 1960s, when a baby (such as myself) came home from the hospital, it was straight to its own bed, own room, blankets, bonnets and bedclothes aplenty and windows wide open to let in all the lovely fresh air, be it a boiling July day or the icy depths of a December night.

Four decades of scientific research later, the world has moved on: 'Baby must must *must* sleep in your room for the first six months,' counselled the antenatal instructor before the birth.

Many of the other mums have taken not the blindest bit of notice, confident to do what works for them, regardless of 'the rules'. But as I have said, being old school and still treating every morsel of advice as gospel, naturally I aim to obey this to the letter.

However, we have fallen foul of logistics: four months in, the baby seems to have doubled in length and is now too big for her crib. We do have a cot – it's just that we can't get it out through her bedroom door and in through ours.

'Time for her own room,' says my husband.

But I fret about disobeying orders, and also worry that sending my wee one out into the world (or at least the room next door) at such a tender age might be too much. (For me.)

For some reason, many of my younger counterparts find this hugely amusing, having reclaimed their boudoirs from the off. But this does not change the fact that I am not ready to let her go and the separation anxiety kicks in.

In the end, we compromise: an air mattress on the floor of the baby's room and I move in with her instead. Just for a few days, but it helps to ease the transition, even if it does also make me a figure of fun for weeks to come.

Now that we are well into our mothering, the range of topics of conversation at our regular gatherings has expanded; it's no longer just poo (colour, texture and frequency thereof) that we discuss over endless tea and biscuits. No – we have finally managed to move away from matters faecal to subjects as diverse and entertaining as car seats, cradle cap and contraception.

Only one person admits to having 'done it' yet. Most look vaguely horrified at the idea of wasting precious bed time by doing anything except sleeping. And when I ask around, this attitude does seem to be pretty much par for the course with, 'I like the idea of it, but if it's a toss-up between that and half an hour's kip, it's no contest,' being the most typical response, regardless of age. As one 30-something friend says, 'Thank goodness my husband is being so good about the fact I have no interest; I was worried that abstinence wouldn't make the heart grow fonder.'

Nonetheless, although my own outlook doesn't seem to differ from the rest, a couple of the older mums I talk to seem to have embraced chastity with such verve that they are in danger of making Cliff Richard look like a floozy.

'Your sex drive is bad enough after having kids,' says one. 'Then just when I thought I might be able to get back in the groove, along comes the menopause and it's back to, "Please, not tonight, I've got a headache and I really need to finish crocheting this lovely lilac toilet roll cover." Not a winning combination for the libido.'

As for me, the very idea of bedroom antics makes me aware that at this particular juncture I may not be at my most alluring, and that considerable effort is needed to get anywhere close to being a femme fatale. Even with the lights off.

Given the fact that I was born a decade before the rest of my antenatal group, I have felt justified in using my age as an excuse for not shaping up as speedily as the rest. But suddenly it appears to be en vogue to 'do' late motherhood and now a whole load of 40-something celebrities have blown my cover by looking immaculate – for all the world to see – within days of giving birth.

Iman, Halle Berry, Madonna – they pop out a baby one minute and it's back to supermodelling or global superstarring the next, with not so much as an excess pound to their names.

Nicole Kidman is the latest star to do the dirty. I figure that maybe I can turn this to my advantage and fire off an email to her agent:

Dear Nicole Kidman

Like you, I have given birth for the first time in my early 40s.

I have been inspired by how amazing you look after the experience. I do not look amazing in the least and would greatly value any tips.

I am writing a book about my experiences of what the doctors (certainly in the UK) describe as 'older motherhood' and so any advice would be hugely appreciated – particularly if I have to make any appearances to publicise it. I am running out of time.

With grateful thanks ...

I do not get a reply.

In the hope that I can still receive wisdom from a top celebrity source, I forward my request on to Halle Berry and Emma Thompson.

In the meantime, I simply try to walk a little more and eat a little less and hope for the best instead. But exercising restraint is not as simple as I'd hoped: as far as I can tell, 'maternity leave' seems to be a synonym for 'social whirl', as we mums bounce from one play date to the next, dangling lurid soft toys at the babies and stuffing ourselves with copious, copious amounts of cake.

Anxious to show prowess in something, I switch on the oven, pull on my pinny and bake for all I am worth. Sponges and sables, cup cakes and croissants. I whip egg whites and beat butter cream till my arms ache with the effort and every surface of the kitchen is covered with cooling patisserie.

But with the cachet comes calories; oh so many calories. And while my audience is appreciative, I realise that perhaps this is where I am going wrong and very possibly one of Nicole's top tips may be not to seek solace in sultana cookies.

Stepping away from the stove and renouncing any ambition to become the next Nigella Lawson does, at least, allow me more time to pursue other activities.

I flirt with the idea of trying out one of the new baby-and-buggy fitness classes that seem to be all the rage –

although nervous at the thought of displaying my disappointing dearth of fitness in public, I figure it may be wise to find out more before enrolling.

And so it is that the baby and I take up position in a rhododendron bush to witness an awe-inspiring procession of pram-pushers march, lunge and dip their way around the park, dripping sweat, co-ordination and competence in equal measure.

We don't return.

On the bright side, this does mean that I get more time to hang out with old friends, though many of my contemporaries have teenagers and tweenagers, so finding activities to suit all ages can have its moments. But there are positives too. They get to tell me where they went wrong – and so I get to learn from their slip-ups (and make a whole bunch of new ones of my very own instead).

Often, my friends' kids find having a teeny one around a great novelty, and the baby revels in being entertained by a succession of prepubescent girls all cooing, oohing and aahing, just as I remember doing at that age.

When I ask around, it is clear that there are blips though. One friend – a single mum at 43 – tells me: 'Most of my old mates have been brilliant – although I'm not invited on joint holidays, as they've admitted they don't want a young child around. The irony is that I wasn't invited on joint holidays when their kids were small either – as then I was single and childless. And that hurt too! So I end up hanging out with my new, younger friends – despite the age difference between us.'

I am standing rather too close to another when I make my enquiries – with hindsight it would have been safer to light the blue touch paper and retire … to another country. 'YES, YES, YES,' she bellows. 'This is the *really* hard bit. My daughter's godmother keeps saying, "I just wish we could have done this together." Aaaaargh … '

As for me? In many ways I've been lucky. And I've certainly found one massive plus: every time we visit friends or family with bigger kids we come away with bags and bags of toys and clothes that they're now done with. So one definite advantage of waiting to start your family is that you get the best-dressed kid in town who thinks that every day is Christmas.

But is there a downside? Hell, yes.

I have had to endure more than a decade of my mates' conversations about nappies and nurseries when I was still into theatre, cinema, books, concerts … Now I want to talk about nappies and nurseries and all they say is, 'Do you remember? Seems so long ago – couldn't face going back to that after all these years. Far too old.'

Er … thanks.

But then nights out with the new, young 'baby friends' have their moments too. One tuts loudly and disapprovingly during a who-does-the-cooking conversation, when I contribute the fact that my husband is the Johnny to my Fanny. My flustered explanations on the merits of Ms Craddock and her sidekick draw a total blank from those who hitherto believed that life BD (Before Delia) was nothing more than a load of cavemen roasting up dinosaurs over open fires. And similarly, my assertion that *Pogles Wood* was the *Peppa Pig* of its day is apparently delivered in Esperanto, judging by the bewildered expressions all round.

But this clash of culture is just one of many, many things that no one thinks to warn you about.

Sure, any pregnancy book will tell you that a multitude of things lies in store for those who are with child. A daunting list, perhaps, given that piles, varicose veins and constipation seemed to be the recurring themes in every tome my friends laid their hands on. But on most fronts, I guess I got lucky, so I shouldn't complain.

But there's another thing that no manual cares to mention – the fact that the second your stomach starts to swell, you become fair game for passing comment from the world, his wife and his second cousin once removed. It is almost as though a doctrine has been issued from on high:

And verily, it has been decreed that any person who crosses your path has divine right to pass judgment upon mother and/or child.

Tact and sensitivity fly straight out of the window. And in the same way that women appear to be fair game for public comment during pregnancy, so it continues after the birth, the focus of the ribald remarks simply switching to the child instead – comments like, 'Hasn't she got a big round face? Just like you.' (It's the neighbour again. I Google 'estate agents' the minute I get home.)

I wonder – would you walk up to a teenager in the street and say, 'Sorry about the acne, love; give it a couple of years and it'll pass'? No, I didn't think so. And yet people I have never seen before in my life now stop me in Tesco to tut at my infant offspring's milk spots, shaking their heads sagely, while muttering things like, 'What a shame.'

Still, on the plus side, I have become quite the authority on the interpretation of the backhanded compliment. Allow me to demonstrate:

What They Say	What They Mean
Oh, isn't she bonny?	She's fat.
How old? Oh, she looks older!	She's fat.
Look at those cheeks!	She's fat.
Isn't she big for her age?	She's fat.
Ooh, aren't you chubby?	She is FAT and what on earth are you feeding her?

Note: just for the record, let me state that a) she really isn't and b) I am following recommended guidelines to the letter, thank you very much.

I am learning not to take people's parlance at face value, but it is becoming ever-more apparent that there's nowt so queer as folk.

The other day my girl, dressed head to toe in fuchsia, was ambushed by a posse of blue-rinsed octogenarians.

'What a lovely little fellow,' cooed one.

'What's his name?' enquired another.

We duly replied.

'What a funny name for a boy,' their puzzled response.

As one who is still scarred from being called 'sonny' at the age of seven (and I was wearing a skirt at the time), I figure that despite my aesthetic objections, we're going to have to go with powder pink and frills until she grows bosoms large enough to allay any ambiguity.

But I am discovering the good side too: the times when complete strangers stop in the street to admire my daughter's big blue eyes or her heart-stopping smile. Best of all, perhaps, a recent stroll in the park during which a three-year-old boy scooted past at great speed, then reversed for a quick, 'Hello, cute baby,' before wheeling off again into the distance. Two foot nothing he might have been, but he sure put a smile on this proud mother's face.

CHAPTER 5

6–9 MONTHS

Six months in and there are gourmet feasts aplenty being prepared in our house. Trouble is, none of them are for me.

Suddenly, it's solids time and consequently I am puréeing everything in sight, including the TV remote, next door's cat and the sofa (though I'm not entirely sure that the latter is actually included in Gina's otherwise comprehensive guide to first-stage weaning).

Day One, and the baby looks baffled to see a dollop of white goo heading towards her mouth ... Day Two, and she is grabbing us by the arm to shove that spoon in as fast as she can.

The kitchen becomes a hive of industry as every day I peel, chop, steam and mush, filling ice-cube tray after ice-cube tray with fruits, vegetables and pulses of every hue, ready for freezing, bagging and labelling.

I have lists and spreadsheets and, suddenly, my life appears to have been taken over by frozen food and I start to feel like Captain Birdseye, albeit with slightly less facial hair. Nonetheless, I find myself making a mental note to check eBay for some suitable naval attire to complete the look. In the meantime, I content myself with dancing around the kitchen shouting, 'Yee ha, me hearties, look out for the grey bits in other fish fingers,' and checking out Annabel Karmel's copious recipes for cod.

Soon, however, this frenzied activity overload begins to take its toll, and just a month after entering this weaning wonderland, I'm beyond exhausted and can barely get off the sofa. I blame my age (again) until, on Remembrance Sunday, I am humbled by the fact that three men, aged 112, 110 and 108 respectively, can make it to the Cenotaph when I cannot even nip round the corner to Tesco. Suitably shamed, I pull on my pinny and it's back to the kitchen.

On the bright side, at least my extra efforts prove worthwhile: be it pear, pea or purée de lentilles et d'herbes (aka savoury mush) the baby necks it down in one, which is, at least, a comfort, as our own culinary needs have now been tossed into the darkest corner where they lie forgotten under a pile of increasingly stale biscuit crumbs, two odd socks and an ever-growing spider's web … At least until my husband returns from work.

'What's for dinner?' he asks. Met with a blank stare and a shrug of the shoulders he rifles through the freezer, only to discover that all that is on offer is cubes, cubes and more cubes. True, for a toothless infant this might constitute a veritable feast – but for an adult I can see that it may be rather less appealing.

I get creative. 'See? Let's take two cubes of leek and potato, two of carrot. We can chuck in a green bean and a sweet potato for colour. A couple of broccolis, a quick blitz in the microwave and hey presto – delicious vegetable soup à la carte.'

He remains unconvinced and slinks off to watch the telly.

I find him in front of a rerun of *Grumpy Old Women*.

'Ha ha ha,' I laugh – partly because it is amusing, but also because I want to show that I may be a terrible housewife but I am, at least, good-humoured and jolly and so still fairly loveable. 'Aren't they so very grumpy? Ha ha ha. Aren't they so very old?'

My husband regards me warily from the other end of the sofa. Let it be said that my other half is a good man, a modern man, a man who knows about hormones and the fact that a large bar of Galaxy can go a long way to avert any argument. However, he is also a wise man, which means it is only when he is halfway out of the front door, en route to the chippy (apparently his only source of sustenance right now), that he points out that not only are several of the women not dissimilar in age to me, but that actually, some of my views make theirs look rather liberal.

Oh woe, woe and thrice woe. I can delude myself no longer. I am old and I am grumpy. I am the person I swore I would never become. One who says, 'Can you turn that down a bit?' or, 'Ooh, they don't do proper tunes any more like they did in my day.' One who describes anything from Top Shop as 'with it'?

It would seem that I am not, as I have tried to believe, immune to the passage of time. And I must come to terms with the fact that I am not the hip, young, trendy mother that I had always imagined myself to be either.

Now I think about it, I must admit that it is true that most evenings you will find me on the sofa, TV control in one hand and a half-eaten bag of Revels in the other. But it still comes as a shock to realise that my days of raving are, apparently, over; and that at the tender age of eight months, my daughter gets invited to more parties than I do.

*

The festive period is upon us.

The baby celebrates by learning to crawl and sprouting a couple of teeth (yes, they do appear on 25 December and yes, they are her two front teeth – now try getting that little Spike Jones classic out of your head …).

I suffer my first chocolate-orange-related injury of the season after underestimating the solidity of the segments when they're all stuck together and tapping (with a view to unwrapping) on my knee with rather too much force. To add insult to said injury, after all this effort I discover that it doesn't even count as one of my five a day.

I figure that a little romance may be what we're missing and spend a happy hour cooking up an elaborate seduction scene involving candlelight, soft music, fancy food and slinky lingerie. (I am thinking 'perhaps a silky peignoir?' until I realise that I'm not actually sure what a peignoir is – though the Danielle Steele phase I went through in the late 80s would suggest that it's something quite essential to any racy overnight activity.) But then a little voice in my head whispers, 'You've only ever worn baggy pyjamas. Aren't you going to be a figure of fun in a lacy cami or the like? And that's before you factor in the Caesarean overhang … '

I book a restaurant instead.

Still, it's exciting to be out on a 'date'. We hold hands, order a delicious meal and enjoy feeding each other tempting morsels from the dishes set before us (at least until I get so tipsy on half a glass of wine that my hand–eye co-ordination goes to pot).

The evening flies by – or so we think, until we ask for the bill and discover it's actually only five past nine. Although we have told the babysitter we won't be late, we are far too embarrassed to arrive home little more than an hour after we left.

And so it is that we find ourselves in Tesco, buying black socks for him, a new hole punch for me, some broccoli and a large bag of Minstrels to split between us. And thereby, we happily return to our life on the sofa.

Meanwhile, the rest of the world continues to throw itself wholeheartedly into a whirl of festive fun. Outside the streets are still thronged with revellers, public transport awash with vomiting office workers staggering home from their various jollies, the shops still full of glitter and little black dresses. But this year I have no interest.

It wasn't always so. In fact, back in the day, when I was a young thing – when black ash furniture was all the rage and the average shoulder pad could double as a pillow for an unexpected guest – New Year's Eve was 'An Event'. How times have changed.

This year there are no crisps or vol au vents (or whatever the latest line in party food may be) – just a nice roast dinner. No hordes of merry party-goers – just me, my husband and my mother-in-law. True, the baby would have upped the numbers and brought the average age down a decade or two, but as she is in bed, I guess that would be cheating.

The other new mothers of my acquaintance party the night away, but for me there is no dancing and no DJ: I am in bed with a cup of cocoa before 10.30. And while I look and feel like death the morning after, alas I cannot blame it on copious quantities of booze – Diet Coke being as strong as it got – but on the bad back and the fact that the next-door neighbour decided the early hours would be a fine time to go into labour. (Don't get me wrong – I have nothing against home births per se; I simply wonder whether they should be restricted to those living in detached properties.) I offer my congratulations to the new parents nonetheless.

So a wild introduction to 2009 it is. The baby sleeps, like a baby in fact, while her parents bemoan their advancing years and take a few paracetamol.

As it happens, I don't really mind. While many of my younger friends are lamenting their lack of social life, I figure I've been out pretty much every night for the last

20 years, so it's quite a relief to have an excuse to stay in with a curry and *X Factor* on a Saturday night.

Maybe this is another advantage of older mother-hood: the fact that some of the changes brought about by baby are welcomed with open arms. Certainly many of my friends would agree: 'I have no desire to be doing anything other than raising my son,' says one 40-year-old. 'I don't wish I was going out on the town or off on exotic holidays. Been there, done that. I had quite a hedonistic time in my twenties and got all of that out of my system years ago.'

And I too am happy to be a home bird. So it seems fitting that for the first time in as long as I can remember, I have made a New Year's resolution: to give the whole domestic goddess thing another whirl. I make this choice based on guilt over my poor form during the previous year and, indeed, when I mention my resolve to my husband he asks whether I have a fever and advises perhaps I should lie down for a while.

But contrary to expectation, I give it my best.

It's the weekend, and by lunchtime I have done two lots of washing, popped into Tesco, baked a batch of banana muffins (revolting, as it happens, but you can't fault the effort). I have also cleaned the house, delivered three presents, had coffee with a friend celebrating her birthday, washed and dressed the baby and kept her amused … though I am wondering why the song is called 'EASY like a Sunday morning'?

And next stop, a giant Swedish Superstore on the North Circular …

… I have discovered that no matter what you are actually intending to purchase at the outset, a higher force kicks in somewhere between the market place and the food mart bit near the exit (where one gets to browse vast quantities of mini Dime bars, a surprisingly wide range of herrings and an assortment of rather delicious gingery baked goods with names like, 'Klip', 'Klop' and 'Håvanöthåbiscuitörtwo').

Law of Ikea
Thou shalt not depart the building without 200 paper napkins and a large bag of tea lights.

And lo, I do return home laden with unneeded serviettes and miniature candles. And verily, I do descend into flat-pack hell the following morning, as I attempt to assemble our new kitchen table. And thus, I do return to the life of sloth in angst and with a sore thumb.

To make matters worse – and to adhere strictly to the rule that DIY disasters hunt in packs – we have a leak. My husband tackles the problem with gusto, but quickly learns that if the U-bend under the sink breaks and the kitchen floods and you clean up using a load of towels, it is not such a great idea to then wring them out into the sink …

And it all goes downhill from there.

I answer my own phone with a cheery hello (a miracle in itself), only to have an American computer tell me, 'I'm sorry, that was an invalid response.'

The next time it rings, I try a more valid response – only to discover it is my mother-in-law I am telling to eff off.

I order flowers, pack up the baby and head into town, far away from screwdrivers and telephones and American computers.

The baby is very overexcited by the bus ride and fascinated by the delights that the West End has to offer. Her mother is less so: it's sale time and manoeuvring the buggy round the hordes of happy shoppers takes some doing.

To be fair, I do have my eye on some bargains myself, but I am daunted, nay thwarted, by the queues: I can only assume that the people who calculated that China is the most densely populated place on earth have never visited Primark in Oxford Street.

My plan is to buy clothes for the baby. Preferably orange, as I am bored with trying to scrub carrot stains out of everything of any other hue – but alas, it would seem that this year's spring fashion has no place for 'apricot', 'tangerine' or 'flame'.

It's a tricky business this. The poor child has inherited my pallor, so unless I want her to look like an oversized Farley's Rusk, cream, beige and similar neutrals are all out. Things with frills and sparkles are vetoed on aesthetic grounds. And things that button up the back are out for logistical reasons. Tights seem to be either at least a foot too long or so baggy around the ankles that my girl would make Nora Batty look like a top-class lingerie model in comparison. And surely it is cruelty to stick a defenceless round and baldy baby in a frou-frou party dress?

As her arms appear to be a perfectly normal length I am not entirely sure why I have yet to find a sleeve that doesn't need rolling up – then rolling up again. And then there are the things that you are supposed to get over your poor child's head without giving her whiplash in the process. (Removing said clothing is even worse, if you want to stop short of decapitation; the scissors have been pressed into emergency action on more than one occasion.)

I do not want my child slathered head to toe in Disney, nor do I want her to look as though she's eight months going on 18; until she is old enough to argue the merits of crop tops and skin-tight leggings for herself we'll be steering well clear. Everything with poppers seems to unpop at an inopportune moment.

And so it would appear that despite my efforts we're still stuck with nothing more than a few humble Baby-gros and one very lovely, fluffy (but still too big) Boden jacket that I found in the sale.

By now, the baby has begun to pick up on my shopping angst and has started to grizzle. But fortunately, here, in the midst of the bustling capital, everyone is far too busy going about their business/ripping off tourists/dodging long, red bendy buses to cast so much as a second glance at a frazzled 40-something mum with a badly dressed babe in tow, so there's something to be thankful for.

My mate Ruby, who has moved to the country, tells me a very different story though:

'In a trendy London suburb I never thought twice about my age. Now, by the sea, I've had a real wake-up call. Suddenly, everywhere I look there are kids pushing prams.

'Last week I went to a comedy club in Dover. One of the comedians, a Londoner with one of the most acerbic tongues I have ever heard, threw the "Who has kids?" question into the audience. A giggling gaggle of girls having a great time laughed, and someone put their hand up. She looked like a small child herself, and the comedian started bantering with her. She had two kids – he looked visibly surprised that this young thing could have children. Then she announced that they were one … and seven! It was the first time the comedian was lost for words all evening! I was sitting there just trying to work out the maths! What a difference 70 miles have made for me as an older mum.'

But that's not to say that there aren't occasionally issues for us London lasses of a certain age. And this is not helped by yet another wave of stories about older motherhood hitting the papers, and I begin to wonder whether a total news blackout might be the only way for me to retain any sort of composure.

One paper's asking me how I will cope with teenage sulks when I'm in my 50s … Badly, I imagine, but judging by my contemporaries who started young and are facing this now, in their 30s and 40s, that's how it works anyway isn't it, whatever your age?

Another report (and another opportunity for my hackles to rise still further) points out that around half of today's older first-time mums have needed help to conceive. Yes, I know, I've read the statistics – but is that really anybody's business but their own? Unless these women are mugging nubile 20-somethings at zebra crossings and bashing them on the head before whipping out their eggs and leaving them barren by the wayside, is this really such a crime?

Apparently so, according to an article which then asks, 'Would *you* want to handle hot flushes at the same time as dealing with a pubescent prima donna?'

At our next girls' night out, yet another news story means there is only one topic of conversation.

This time, a piece in an august medical journal has said that older mums are more prone to cancer, heart attacks and depression and describes the 'epidemic' of pregnancy in middle age as a 'threat to public health'.

I am riled enough to let my starter go cold, which is saying a lot. And I am not alone.

'It's all very well to say that the optimum age for giving birth is somewhere between 20 and 35 but if you haven't met the right person by then what exactly are you meant to do? Pick some random passer-by just to impregnate us before our use-by date?' bellows Nicola at a volume that unwittingly draws the rest of the restaurant into our heated debate.

'It's an outrage!' harrumphs Kate with such passion that she almost falls off her soap box and causes a woman at a neighbouring table to drop her profiteroles all over the floor.

Indeed we get so carried away with the ins and outs and injustice of it all that we don't even have time to order dessert before closing time – which, frankly, does nothing to improve our ill humour.

But a few days later, a surprise.

Is it? No, surely not … Can this really be an article that brings good news for a change? Indeed, it is.

Hurrah for the piece (which I have photocopied and used as wallpaper in my hallway) that tells us we 'older' mums are less likely to be dragged down by the menopause than our younger counterparts.

Hurrah for our stored oestrogen and its long-lasting and beneficial effects on our muscles, bones and nerves.

And three cheers for the fact we (apparently) are too busy taming toddlers to have any time to worry about thinning hair or nasty night sweats. (Although a dismayed 50-something chum with a 12-year-old daughter says, 'Really – are you sure that's not a load of bollocks? I've found the menopause a bloody nightmare.' … Oh.)

So let us move on and, while we're at it, give a gold star to the researchers involved in the New England Centenarian study showing that women who give birth at 40-plus are four times more likely to live to 100!

See – turns out we might even get to meet our grand-children after all. Not to mention have a telegram from our sovereign to hand down as a family heirloom.

And we're on a roll! In another article are the findings of a survey involving four-year-olds, showing that those born to older mums come out top in tests of their verbal and intellectual ability. All down to our parenting practices apparently, as we are more likely to invest quality time in our kids.

Which, at least, gives me hope for the future.

I like to think that my daughter will look back at her childhood with only cheerful reminiscence and determine that I will do all I can to ensure she has the requisite store of happy memories to carry with her all her life.

I have many happy memories of childhood myself, though the three recollections that always seem to spring straight to mind are these (which, I hasten to add, speak volumes about the vagaries of my brain, rather than any omission on the part of my wonderful parents):

1) I am aged four, dressed in a polyester slacks combo (remember that this is the era of Brentford Nylons, the cusp of the decade of static, and anything made of natural fibres is considered terribly outré – although this does mean that any child born in the late 1960s or early '70s comes with an innate appreciation of the dangers of standing

within a hundred yards of a naked flame, so it's not all bad). My mother is on the phone to a friend. They are talking about a neighbour's smear test – something I do not take on board until many, many years later – but, in any case, I am focusing only on the bit where the neighbour pops to the loo beforehand, then – with only scratchy hard loo paper on offer – fishes around in her handbag for a tissue. When she lies down for the examination and removes her undergarments, the doctor is somewhat baffled to see a set of Green Shield stamps stuck haphazardly over her nether regions.

None of my friends under 40 has ever heard of Green Shield stamps (or scratchy loo paper, for that matter), so nowadays this rather loses something in the telling, but to this day it has left me very wary of any stray adhesive miscellanea about my person in the event that I have to grab a tissue in a lavatorial situation.

2) I am aged eight and have had a day trip to the Lake District with my school friend and her family. I am wearing a C & A trouser suit –

denim flares and denim shirt (worn open as a jacket), each embroidered with a nonchalantly lolling cowboy. We have Quavers for lunch which, for some reason unknown to me, but nonetheless proven on more than one occasion, do not agree with me; and thus it is on the homeward stretch of the M6 that I projectile vomit down the neck of my friend's father (who is driving) and all over the pristine leather interior of his brand new Jag. I also recall far too clearly her mother having to help me strip to my knickers on the hard shoulder and then me asking to move class on the Monday because I am too embarrassed to ever look my friend in the eye again.

3) Back to age four, and it is my brother's second birthday party. As the 'big girl' in a room full of toddlers I am dressed to impress – in another trouser suit, as it happens, this one made of tangerine crimplene with jaunty flares and a sleeveless jacket worn over a white polo. White socks and gold sandals complete the look. Naturally, this is so long ago that the incriminating photographs are in black and white, yet the memory of the

lurid man-made fabrics has not been dulled by time.

I may only be at the beginning of the learning curve that is motherhood, but already these reminiscences have made one thing crystal clear: I must never ever buy my daughter a trouser suit as it will undoubtedly colour all her childhood memories – and not for the better.

Fashion has been pushed down the agenda by the fact the child is on the move and my current concern must therefore be safety measures: things to keep her from falling down stairs, things to keep her from climbing upstairs and things to prevent her from generally heading with magnetic force towards any remotely dangerous object at the speed of Jenson Button.

I have hitherto eschewed the bulk of infant para-phernalia, not really seeing the need for a wipe warmer (unless you store your wipes in the freezer I guess, in which case you are certainly likely to fall into the cate-gory of 'more money than sense'). Then there are bolsters to stop one's baby rolling over when it can't actually roll over yet, in any case. And those brightly coloured, teeny tiny knee pads to 'protect' those little legs as they start to crawl – presumably over the shards of glass and nails that one generally has lying about the house, rather than your bog-standard carpet.

Somehow, we have also managed to live without the gift that an American friend offered (threatened?) to send: arm-shaped pillows (complete with fingers) which come with the promise of comforting and protecting your infant by allowing it to feel that there is a 'little bit of you' with him or her at all times. I vetoed this contribution on the grounds that:

a) I want my child to know that there are times when she can cope very nicely on her own, thank you

b) I am not convinced that waking to find oneself cradled by a pair of severed/stuffed hands is ideal in terms of formative experience and I do not want a precious friendship to be destroyed by arguments over who is to blame for the child's traumatic flashbacks in later life, and

c) an alternative gift (along the lines of the more standard soft toy/fleecy blanket/rattle shaped like a frog) would work out much cheaper than the years of therapy I would otherwise be obliged to sue her for.

I admit that even I was seduced by a suction bowl that was, according to the blurb, meant to stick firmly to the table in all conditions up to and including earthquakes no greater than 5.7 on the Richter scale, but which, in actual fact, the child managed to knock flying within a nano second. And thus I learned my lesson.

But now? Now I find myself browsing kiddie catalogues like a good 'un, weighing up which of the thousands of baby safety accessories I simply cannot live without and trying to second guess what my little Evil Knievel is going to attempt next.

As the child hurls herself head first on to the terrazzo floor yet again, it seems that top of the list should be a stair gate. And fast. I am fairly sure that the local mega market sells them, but figure that it is probably wise to ring first to check and thus prevent a wasted journey.

The wasted journey would have been quicker.

Things I get to do while on hold for the customer service desk: paint my toenails; knock up a surprisingly tasty pasta sauce; pick all the fluff off my favourite sweater ...

When I do finally mange to speak to someone, the unenthusiastic assistant goes off to check and informs me that no – the toy section is all out of Stargate. Given that I have clearly explained my needs I do wonder why she would ever have thought that a Stargate Winged Glider Alien Attack Craft might stop a kamikaze baby from falling down the staircase, but rather than waste yet more time on a clearly fated mission, I simply head for Mothercare instead.

As the child has the resolve of an intrepid explorer determined not be thwarted by anything in her path I also buy cupboard locks. Which we cannot work out how to fit. And so we buy a different type. Which we cannot work out how to fit either.

We buy socket covers which we cannot then remove from the sockets (although, on the bright side, this does save us a fortune in electricity because we now can't use any of our appliances. Every cloud, and all that …).

I discover that there are things to put on blinds and things to put on fridges, things to put on doors and things to put on toilets and things to put on cookers. It's an impressive array, though I do wonder how I managed to get through my own childhood in one piece, given I had nothing more than a pram harness and a playpen to keep me from harm.

I ask my mother how she coped in the days before this splendid assortment of safety equipment was invented and she says, 'I told you I would throttle you if you put your fingers in the sockets and it seemed to work.'

The days I grew up in seem so much simpler. There were no computer games, no computers even – and so we played out on our bikes or built dens in the garden. There were no mobile phones, so if we wanted to thank someone properly for a birthday gift (as was the custom in days of yore) we could not text a quick and cursory message, but would be stood over by our mothers as we painstakingly scratched out a whole pile of 'Dear Auntie … ' missives on a selection of flowery notelets (*always* a flowery notelet and always 'Auntie' and 'Uncle', whether you were related or not – the idea of calling a grown-up by their first name being unimaginable to anyone under 18).

Ah yes, in my day people still had antimacassars and black and white tellies and Channels Four and Five were yet to be invented. There was none of your CBeebies or Nick Jr. – just *Mary, Mungo and Midge*, *Andy Pandy* or *Tom and Jerry*, and then only as a treat for eating all your tapioca pudding or feeding next door's budgie while the owners holidayed in exotic climes, such as Southport or Scarborough.

And now (in what must be the surest sign yet that middle age is upon me), whenever I trawl the Internet for information I find myself all nostalgic for my complete set of *Children's Encyclopaedia Britannica*, the fount of all knowledge when I was a nipper, with everything you could ever possibly want or need to know about anything all wrapped up in that distinctive red leatherette binding.

A fuddy-duddy I may be, but I want to sit my girl down with volume seven (aka, if my memory serves me rightly, though quite possibly it doesn't, 'Lions to Moonbeams') and teach her that 'M' is for 'Manners'. I will explain to her that these are things that you don't see so many of nowadays, given that a large proportion died out around the same time as the thrupenny bit and the fad for Parma Violets. But that will not stop us from upholding the traditional values – the pleases and thank yous – in our house. And if that means that forever more she shall be known as 'daughter of the dinosaur', then so be it.

At least I can take comfort in the fact that I am not alone in my mission nor, judging by the many other older mums I meet, the only one who grows wistful for the low-tech simplicity of the 1970s. Indeed, I am gladdened by the fact there seem to be a fair few of us out there and wonder if there should be a collective noun for our merry, if slightly arthritic, band … Perhaps a Zimmer?

CHAPTER 6

9–12 MONTHS

It would appear that I am a medical phenomenon.

With the rapid approach of my birthday, I have examined the last 12 months in great detail and made an important scientific discovery: namely that I am ageing at least seven times faster than any of my contemporaries and must, therefore, conclude that I have mysteriously switched to dog years.

How else can I account for the fact that time has flown so fast?

I catch sight of myself in a mirror and am shocked to find the face staring back at me is 20 years older than it ought to be. (Though the solution to that is obvious. Avoid mirrors.)

But even a fleeting glance at my reflection as I pass a shop window serves to remind me that my first flush of youth is long gone.

As far as I can tell, the main difference between early 20s and early 40s is about a stone and a half. Although there is the whole birthday thing as well …

Acquaintance about to turn 24: 'I am so excited. It's my birthday on Friday. I'm having a party and I just can't wait.'

Chum about to turn 44: 'Oh god, it's my birthday on Friday. How depressing is that? Don't tell anyone will you?'

But this whole ageing business is a funny old thing – and I confess it can leave me slightly baffled.

Read the tabloids when Cherie Blair gave birth at 45, and you'd have thought it was an absolute miracle that someone so utterly ancient could possibly push one out. But when Tony became Prime Minister at 44? The world's press went crazy over his youth.

Yet given the similarities between the two roles – lots of sleepless nights, people telling them how to do their job, a ton of pictures for the family album, immeasurable pride at their achievement (and so on and so forth) – I cannot fathom the reasons for this double standard.

I have asked around and no one seems to be able to come up with anything either, though I do get several diatribes along the lines of, 'How come when people like Michael Douglas or Paul McCartney have babies in their late 50s or even 60s they get nothing but congratulations, but when it's Susan Sarandon or Geena Davis in their late 40s, everyone goes on about it for weeks? Because it's a MAN'S WORLD … '

Perhaps this is the case. Or perhaps it is simply that when it comes to age we are judged – even unwittingly – by our ability to procreate. And if fertility truly is the secret of eternal youth, it's tough luck indeed for the fairer sex, as for us, sowing our seed ad infinitum is not an option. Like it or not, this theory makes us pretty much past it by the time we hit our half century.

Of course, I do understand that in days of yore, even 43 years of wear and tear may well have seen me tucked up in a rocking chair, knitting bootees for my grandchildren. But this is the 21st century and surely times have changed?

Yes, I might have a bad back and rather more wrinkles than I would care for, but I am also financially and emotionally settled – quite a good place to be I'd say, when it comes to starting a family. I have infinitely more patience than I did at 25 or 30 and am happy, rather than frustrated, at the idea of taking a temporary step back from the hustle and bustle of the last couple of decades.

Yes, yes, mid-life may be upon me, but I am no ancient crone. And, truth be told, in this new game of motherhood, in the face of teething, tantrums and the like, age is so often immaterial and I pay it no more heed than the cracked window pane in the porch or the festering jar of pickle at the back of the fridge; that is, it's there – I know it's there – and it's not something that fills me with unfettered joy, but generally, I have more pressing things to consider, such as how to get tickets for the FA Cup Final or did I remember to series link *Peppa Pig*?

I appreciate that I can be slow to move with the times. That even 20-odd years on I still have not learned to call a Marathon a Snickers. That I still think of Cif as Jif and will never be able to see Oil of Olay as anything other than Oil of Ulay (and frankly, if they're only going to change one letter why even bother?). But please understand that I am not entirely stuck in the dim and distant past.

I still have my own hair, I still have my own teeth and hell, I even know who's number one in the hit parade (do they still call it the hit parade?). Surely all is not yet lost?

Here in the UK, with the *average* age of giving birth about to hit 30 for the first time (a figure that is rising year on year), I guess it stands to reason that there have to be a fair few of us geriatrics out there to balance out all the teenage pregnancies that never seem to be out of the papers either.

Sure, the press might make much of those having babies in their 40s – yet among my own established social circle, having a child in the course of your fifth decade is nothing out of the ordinary. Indeed, I have yet to hear any of us new mums say they're too old for this malarkey (though the dads are another matter altogether …).

All the same, it will not have escaped your notice that many of the new friends with whom I mix nowadays *are* young. And while the bond of motherhood draws us together, it becomes ever-more apparent that the generation gap forms a cultural chasm that threatens to divide.

This continues to show itself in many forms.

Now that the baby's a bit older I have realised that gurgling at her mother all day may not be the best in developmental aids. And so, in an attempt to encourage her inner Mozart, I have enrolled for a music group in order that she gets to gurgle at a tambourine and a battered plastic shaker instead.

The babies spend most of their time chewing the instruments and looking jolly, if slightly bewildered. And the mothers throw inhibition to the wind and join together in rousing choruses of all the childhood classics. Those born in the '70s and (how this pains me) the '80s sing joyfully that they are 'merry and bright'. Yet I, child of the '60s, am defiantly, resolutely (and tunelessly) 'merry and gay'.

My new friends are good friends. But they just do not realise that Sheena Easton took the morning train, worked from nine till five and then took another home again. They do not understand that the recent disappearance of Quaker Oat Krunchies is a blow hard to stomach. They did not know *Blue Peter* when John Noakes and Peter Purves (or even Simon Groom) were at the helm. Therefore, they did not enter the Goldie limerick competition in which I was a runner-up. And for them, pounds, shillings and pence is an alien concept.

It is unlikely that any of them could – or indeed would – spend an entire evening bemoaning the fact that the speaking clock appears to have gone American. They do not grieve for the 'third stroke' at which it would have been 'three forty-four precisely', nor lament the passing of the clipped tones that could have come straight from *Brief Encounter*. And thus, I alone mourn the fact that Tinkerbell has just told me that it's 'two six', before asking if I would like my eggs over easy and reminding me to have a nice day. Peter Pan would spin in his grave.

So yes, while I may like to delude myself that I am still 'down with the kids', the evidence would suggest otherwise.

In theory, this cloud should have a silver lining. After all, many an adage would have it that the advancement of years brings with it an enhancement of knowledge, that great age and great wisdom go together like, say, Morecambe and Wise, Cagney and Lacey, rhubarb and custard.

Sure, it may be a while till I'm officially pensioned off, yet two score years and 10 looms ever closer and, whichever way you look at it, my first flush of youth has careered off into the distance to be reunited with Captain Pugwash, the Clangers and a load of Old English Spangles.

On the plus side, however, you would think that this would put me in an excellent position to deal with any questions my daughter may have when she reaches the 'Why?' stage.

True, we are not quite there yet. And while my beloved will chatter happily all day (just like her mother), at the tender age of 10 months her vocabulary is somewhat limited. We're still on the basics – 'pah pah' (panda), 'kyu' (thank you), the obligatory 'mamma' and 'daddad'. Oh, and 'yum yum'. She likes her food. Just like her mother.

Yet if a look can speak a thousand words – albeit some of them still unintelligible – it may be that our pride and joy is already questioning the sagacity of her parents.

'Yes yes,' she says in a glance. 'I know perfectly well what "No" means but explain *why* I cannot pull the grate off the fireplace and watch the coals tumble so tempt-ingly on to the hearth rug?'

Or, 'Does the fact that I am able to undo my own nappies not illustrate great dexterity on my part? So why get so het up about it?'

How time has flown.

In the blink of an eye my mewling newborn has become a child whose curiosity knows no bounds.

My mother looks at her and says, 'It only seems like five minutes since you were that age.'

Given it's actually a large fistful of decades it seems I may be on the spot before I know it. I'd better start swotting.

Even if there is still time for cerebral improvement on my part, I fear that when the wee 'un does learn to string a sentence together she may find her mother lack-ing. I do not see how I am placed to answer all her ques-tions and queries when I still have so many of my own.

Why, for example, does every board book and bath toy in the house teach my daughter that ducks – not ducklings – are yellow? I have never seen a yellow duck. Also, I need to know where Junction three of the M1 is hiding. Plus, who thought that putting coffee creams in Revels was acceptable practice? And why was the woman in front of me in Tesco buying 17 iceberg lettuces … ?

It is a long list.

Perhaps I have simply bucked the trend and got older without getting wiser. I await the 'why' years with trepidation, though I hope that when the time comes I will muddle my way through it like many a parent before me. And I'll learn to accept that there will always be some things that are beyond my ken.

For example, I ask myself daily: how did I get so lucky to have this sweet, funny, eccentric little girl as my daughter?

But then some questions don't need answers.

As my maternity leave draws to an end, I realise I am enjoying my new life too much to return to a career that will take me away from my daughter five long days a week, not to mention evenings, weekends and obligatory all-nighters.

I have spent 20 years working in an industry where experience is increasingly no match for youthful enthusiasm, and bright, successful women fall by the wayside in droves after they start their families and try to attain that elusive life/work balance. I am not surprised when someone tells me that it has been voted top in terms of worst careers for working mums.

And so I agonise over career changes and struggle to marry my dreams of doing something new and exciting with my desire to spend more time at home. I grapple with the emotional trauma of stepping out of one career at the top and entering a new one at the bottom and spend most evenings wailing with frustration.

Many of my younger friends rush happily back to their jobs, anxious to make partner, to climb the ladder of success before their childbearing absence loosens a rung on the ladder of success.

But I am 10 years farther down the line, 10 years farther along the mortgage payments, and feel less urgency to return to fighting the battles on the front line full time.

Other friends opt to take career breaks, waiting until their children start school before heading back to the workplace. But for me, this is not an option. Starting over at the age of almost 50 would just be too big a mountain to climb.

And so I struggle on, trying to marry motherhood with ambition, financial security with family values, as I search for my new career.

I am offered a month's work in an august publishing house which I accept only marginally less tearfully than Gwyneth Paltrow on receipt of her Oscar.

I am anxious to make a good impression and the ironing board is brought out of retirement on the eve of my first day.

It is a culture shock to be out in the real world, but I like what I see. Here, having kids is the norm, and barely anyone works a five-day week. However, I grow increasingly perturbed by my inability to remember people's names which, coupled with an appalling sense of direction, makes working in a new (and very large) office somewhat testing.

The department head calls me in for a meeting and I am keen to impress. Part-way through the conversation, I decide to make notes – a move that proves to be my undoing, as I brandish my pen with a flourish, only to discover that it is actually a breadstick in my hand.

And it is not the only time that I run into trouble with baked goods that first day. At lunchtime I select the crusty baguette without taking into account the consequences of consuming it in the quietest open-plan office in Europe. Every bite resonates across an entire floor and a hundred heads turn sharply in my direction. Given that I am ravenous, however, I am loath to lose my lunch and consider how long it will take me to suck the sandwich noiselessly – about three hours, as it turns out.

For the rest of the week I eat soup, bananas and marshmallows.

My new routine is very different from the one I have known before.

8am old life: rise slowly and enjoy leisurely bath and breakfast before leaving for work. 8am new life: quick shower – done. One load of washing – done. Second load already on. Dishwasher emptied. Baby changed and fed. Baby changed again. Lunch and tea sorted. Paper-work dealt with. Go to work for a rest …

Although I am loving my return to the workplace, there is something rather strange about being the new girl when you are in your 40s. I feel slightly fraudulent assuming the role of an ingénue: I've had more than a decade of running teams of tens of people, budgets of hundreds of thousands of pounds. And now I am asking anyone if they'd like a cup of tea and fretting over the number of sugars I was meant to put in the milky one and whether the herbal bag is meant to stay in or out? Oh – and finding my way back from the kitchen …

In my previous existence, I would fly round the world to interview celebrities and presidents. I might lunch with John Lydon, grab a drink with Paul Whitehouse, chat about football with Clive Anderson. There were World Cups, and parties and premières and … And now I'm the spare pair of hands on a potty-training photo shoot and cleaning up the urine (and worse) of a weeping toddler who really isn't taking stage direction very well.

Making this change may well have been my idea, but as keen as I am to make it happen – and I am, I am, I am – it's going to take some getting used to.

Certain I can't be the only mid-life mum to have found herself in this position, I ask around to see how others have coped. And sure enough – a former colleague finds herself in the very same boat:

'TV is a young person's game,' she tells me. 'And the industry does not really accommodate the demands of family life. Trouble is, I've done it for ever and I have no idea what to do next. And I'm a bit old to start out at the very bottom all over again … '

'Ah, you'll get there', comforts a friend sensing my angst and feeding me large slabs of lemon drizzle cake as consolation. 'It doesn't really matter what you do. Just make the most of the time you're at work, make the most of the time you're at home, and it will all come out in the wash'.

A temperate mix of career and kids does sound pretty good to me – and so I relax, enjoy and, as the weeks go by, discover another advantage of working too: the fact that I suddenly have things to talk about other than weeing and weaning. Now that I get to read the paper on the train every morning, I am soon back up to speed with what's going on in the outside world and I congratulate myself on being able to hold my own on important matters of state, such as Susan Boyle's admission to the Priory and Katie Price's love life.

I meet a woman at a dinner party who is, apparently, charmed by my take on the arts and laughs uproariously every time I say anything, declaring to the rest of the table that I am 'delightfully lowbrow'.

I am guessing that this is not a compliment. So it pains me to admit that her own (slightly higher-brow) opinions on women and work are actually (and unexpectedly) fairly sound.

'Being an older mother is actually very positive from an economic point of view,' she intones. 'They have spent longer working and paying taxes and are less likely to depend on state assistance because of this.'

See? I am positively a hero. I knew it …

My contract at an end, it's back to bits of freelance work and trying to work out what I really do want to be when I grow up.

It is finally starting to sink in that this 'having-it-all' lark may be tougher than I thought. With the aid of a Venn diagram (it's only taken 40 years, but I have finally found a use for these ...), I calculate that I can hold down a full-time job *and* spend all day with the baby – as long as I give up sleep. I am not so sure I'm going to make it work.

As a short-term measure, I end up working part time from home. I miss being part of a team, but the arrangement does have its plusses, such as being able to wear a tracksuit and eat cold sausages, while researching umbilical cord stumps: Waynetta Slob meets Penelope Leach.

In the meantime, the baby is changing so fast that I don't want to miss a minute with her. She has learned to clap and wave and eat soil. She can say 'night night' and climb the stairs and blow kisses.

She has fallen in love for the first time (and, fortunately, Bear loves her back again), and every time she says 'Mamma' my heart melts just a little more.

I have learned a lot over these last 12 months, although it is mainly by trial and error, given that I have – to no avail – searched high and low for a manual specifically aimed at the older mother. I can only conclude that others in my position have also been forced to make this mysterious, rather creaky journey without guidance.

With this in mind, a pregnant friend (who, like me, is not exactly in the first flush of youth) asks me to prepare a handbook of my findings vis-à-vis the combination of middle age and new motherhood. Naturally, I am only too happy to oblige.

A is for 'ancient'. This is how you will feel when you hear the woman next to you at the antenatal clinic discussing her plans for her 20th birthday party.

B is for 'burp'. Something that merits as much praise when emitted by one's newborn as it does disdain when emanating from one's spouse. It is also for 'breasts' (and may I take this opportunity to advocate underwiring if you hope to keep them positioned anywhere above your waist).

C is for 'car seat'. Unless you have the bone density of a 25-year-old, do not even consider lugging your baby around in one (see also 'S'). Useful tip: C is also for 'calcium supplements'.

D is for 'doggy'. Note that it is wise to remember your audience and reserve such diminutives for conversing with the under-twos. You really don't want to be discussing 'horsies' and 'moo cows' with your boss.

E is for 'energy' and also for 'eBay'. Alas, I have discovered that you cannot purchase extra supplies of the former on the latter.

F is for 'forgetfulness'. You may have been the most organised person on the planet in a former life – but this does not mean you will avoid the curse of Nappy Brain. **Note**: I have found it useful to have one's name and phone number written on the back of one's hand for reference.

G is for 'girth'. Alas the combination of age and Caesarean section will do this no favours.

H is for 'hair band'. Even if your baby is a girl, do not allow it to sport a hair band unless the child actually has hair. Otherwise this is a Very Bad Thing.

I is for 'I love you'. Which you will never tire of saying. It is also for 'ice cream', which you will never tire of eating (refer to 'G' before purchasing excess quantities of Ben and Jerry's).

J is for 'journey'. It does not matter how long your voyage by train or plane – your child will only fall asleep seven minutes before you arrive. Do not bother buying any magazines to read en route.

K is for 'kak kak'. This is the noise that ducks make (according to my daughter).

L is for 'leisure time' and 'lie in'. Ha ha ha ha ha. L is also for 'lingerie' (and perhaps worth mentioning a cautionary note: maternity bras and/or size 16 'pregnancy' pants do not, apparently, count).

M is for 'mucus' (specifically nasal). Your baby will appear to have an endless supply. Each wipe will induce great misery from said child and so the vicious circle continues …

N is for 'nappies' (specifically dirty ones). Everyone tells you that when it's your own baby they are 'fine'. They are lying.

O is for 'osteopath'. See also 'C' and 'S'.

P is for 'play dates'. I have said this before and I shall say it again: you should be aware that these always involve copious calories. When Marie Antoinette said, 'Let them eat cake', she was actually referring to NCT reunions. 'P' is also for 'purée' and 'posset' (see 'steam cleaning').

Q is for 'questions'. You will have an endless list. This is normal.

R is for 'rolling'. You will be as pleased as punch when your baby first masters this ancient art. You will be less pleased when they insist on displaying their new-found skills while you are attempting a nappy change.

S is for 'slipped disc' (see also 'C'). It is also for 'steam cleaning' (see also 'P').

T is for 'toy envy'. In a previous life, you may have suffered from 'car envy' or 'house envy'. Now you will find that the absolute 'must haves', the greatest objects of desire, are made from brightly coloured plastic. You will devour the Toys R Us catalogue with a fervour formerly reserved for *Elle Decoration*.

U is for 'unbridled joy'. I cannot quantify how much our daughter has brought into our lives. It makes Manchester United winning the Treble pale into insignificance. Which is saying a *lot*.

V is for 'vision'. Which can behave strangely after a prolonged lack of sleep (although I admit that this may be, in part, because I am reaching an age where I need reading glasses but am not yet prepared to admit it). 'Oh look, horsies', I cooed to my daughter as my husband drove us North up the M1 and I spotted a van's distinctive signage. It was only as we passed that I realised it actually read 'Hovis'.

W is for 'weaning' (see also 'steam cleaning'). Your shopping list will consist solely of butternut squash and carrots and you will no longer laugh at Auntie Edie for leaving the plastic cover on her sofa.

X is for 'expert'. A large proportion of your elderly relatives will fall into this category when it comes to bringing up baby. Simply nod sagely and with gratitude at all proffered instruction, then discard as necessary.

Y is for 'yes'. Ensure that this is your immediate response when anyone else offers to cook dinner.

Z is for 'zip it'. All too soon comes a time when it is wise to keep shtum in certain situations. A lesson learned recently after being cut up by another driver. My immediate reaction was to mutter, 'Cow.' Loudly. 'Moooooo,' said a little voice in the back ...

CHAPTER 7

12–18 MONTHS

My baby is one.

Over the last 12 months I have watched my teeny, baldy bundle of joy blossom into a tousle-haired toddler – although I admit that I use the latter term loosely, as we're not exactly overdoing it on the ambulatory front at the moment.

I have learned to marvel at a whole new world, as seen through the eyes of a little girl who's got joie de vivre down to a very fine art. A world in which a glimpse of a chicken ('Cluck CLUUUUCK') elicits as much excitement as a winning lottery ticket. Where the very sight of a tub of soapy liquid produces joyful squawks of, 'Bubbles, bubbles, Mama.' Where a grey rubber doorstop or an empty plastic bottle can afford every bit as much fun as the best that Hamleys has to offer.

It's a good place to be.

But at the same time, I have realised how little I really knew about parenthood – and I have learned how to perform U-turns at a speed that would leave Usain Bolt standing.

'I'm not having the house turn into one big play-room,' the pregnant me insisted to anyone who would listen, mindful of the fact that everyone I knew with children had gradually submerged under piles of gaily coloured plastic.

Now, as I trip over yet another ersatz animal on my way to the sink, pick up shapes and cups of every imaginable hue, move a pile of fluffy rabbits off the sofa so a guest can sit down, I can see that idealism and reality are very different things.

Where once I was adamant that no daughter of mine would conform to type, now I open the wardrobe and am confronted by a sea of pink. But hey – what's a little volte-face between friends?

As I pull back the curtains (pink, naturally) to see the dawning of a new day, I find myself marvelling at how fast the year has flown by.

My baby is one. Who'd have thought it?

The first birthday is, of course, a milestone for any mother. The first birthday party? More of a millstone methinks. It's that pesky aspiration v. actuality thing again.

At one, we had deemed our daughter too young for any large-scale revelry. A party was pointless, we said. Perhaps a little family tea …

So how we came to have a houseful of tiddlers running riot, scattering crumbs near and far and hitting each other over the head with Mr Whoozit and a selection of tambourines, jingle bells and maracas, I am not entirely sure. Although, on a positive note, at least I was afforded the opportunity to plan a birthday feast to put Annabel Karmel to shame.

For days on end, my mind ran away with utopian notions of pinwheel sandwiches, fluffy, light-as-a-feather cupcakes in the shape of every farmyard creature you can think of, assorted fruit snacks cleverly crafted into intricate statuettes and perhaps a breadstick reconstruction of the Eiffel Tower. Yes, my fantasies carried me to a place far beyond my artistic capabilities, but I happily shoved reality firmly to one side.

That is, until I double-checked my diary. And discovered that my daughter's big day fell slap bang in the middle of Passover.

For those who are not familiar with this festival, I shall summarise thus: Moses decides to leave Egypt. Pharaoh says, 'No.' Moses gathers his people and they make a run for it, leaving before their bread has had time to rise. Consequently, for eight days each year thereafter, unleavened bread (aka matzo – think cream cracker meets balsa wood) is de rigueur and anything else made with yeast, flour or any other grain is firmly off the menu.

I admit that this version of events is somewhat concise – but I am sure it is adequate to explain why my dreams of culinary glory evaporated in a haze of cardboard crumbs. The bunny-shaped sandwich cutter that slid so smoothly through a slice of freshly baked bread simply reduced the unleavened variety to rubble. And then there was the further stress of trying to stop a load of toothless infants from choking on matzo, which, trust me, adds a whole new dimension to any festivities.

I did my best. Though my head is still swimming from cutting 200 mini marshmallows into thirds and sticking them – one by one – on to the (flour-free) cake, in order to create 'wool' for the sheep (a paschal lamb if ever there was one?).

And yet I am already thinking about next year. Should we go for a panda? Perhaps a fairytale castle? Or maybe we'll keep the Passover theme going strong with a reconstruction of the parting of the Red Sea. It's amazing what you can do with a bit of food colouring if you put your mind to it ...

Plans for future festivities are put on hold, for suddenly I have bigger fish to fry.

A new obsession appears to be permeating the ranks like a particularly nasty bout of norovirus. One minute everyone is happily pulling party poppers and celebrating first birthdays – the next they are consumed with angst, taking to their beds and vomiting constant streams of panic about schools.

Despite the fact that there are still a couple of years until we are even allowed to *apply* for places, it seems that the very mention of the phrase 'catchment area' now causes instant mass hysteria, arm waving and fainting – a bit like being at a Beatles gig, but with slightly more modern haircuts and no one called Ringo.

The cosy chats about Baby Gap, finger food and sleep patterns are sadly no more. Now at every mummy meet-up I am bewildered by bombardments of Ofsted this and key-stage that until I have no idea what to think about anything.

It is nearly four decades since I started primary school and a chat with a teacher friend confirms that everything has changed. It seems that gone are the days of the greaseproof loo paper which was about as absorbent as a sheet of shiny plastic and led to many a sticky-handed child becoming a pariah in the playground.

Gone are the days of rulers across the knuckles and the threat of the headmaster's cane. Gone are the days when PE was done – boy or girl – with your vest tucked into your pants, the look topped off by a pair of greying plimsolls.

Maybe this education thing was always as competitive as an Olympic final and my memories of a more innocent age, where no one lied about addresses, rented flats they never actually set foot in or stabbed their next-door neighbours for living 0.0001 of a mile closer to a desirable educational establishment, are coloured by the mists of time – and yet I think not.

In recent months, the papers have been filled with tales of cheating parents who've been flouting the system so flagrantly that it's little wonder they get found out. And while (to my knowledge) no one that I know personally has ever stooped as low as breaking the law, one cannot deny that these are crazy times.

I know of no two-year-old in the 1960s or early '70s who went to nursery to do anything but paint, sing songs about rabbits and wet their knickers, and yet a friend's daughter has already been offered a place in a 'crammers' class before she's reached her second birthday. I know three-year-olds who have tutors to get them through entrance 'exams', toddlers whose every waking minute is filled with flash cards.

I want to shout, 'Don't panic, Mr Mainwaring ... ' (except no one would get the cultural reference) ' ... it never did us any harm to go to the local infants', where everyone walked to school and then went home and played in the garden without worrying about completing a part-time degree in brain surgery before they were seven, and still managed to grow up and become teachers and doctors and lawyers and ... '

But perhaps it is time for me to stop harking back to the days when a Jacob's Orange Club was the height of luxury, when the Clangers were the hip young things of children's TV and when in-car entertainment meant nothing more than an eight-track of Leo Sayer's *Greatest Hits* – over and over (and over) again.

Perhaps I must move with the times, get real and work out what to do with the rest of them. As long as it's within the law – of course. Oh hell – where are those Ofsted reports?

And so, like the rest, I duly ingest the necessary information, although once I have established that there is not a thing I can do for another 12 months, I shelve the panic and continue in my efforts to navigate my way through the voyage of discovery that is motherhood. And I'll need all the energy I can muster, for it seems that every new day exposes another new gap in my knowledge.

True, that until a year or so ago, my hands-on experience of babies could be neatly summarised as 'very little', but nonetheless, I figured I had them sussed. Sleep, poo, cry, food, gurgle, sleep, poo and so on and so forth.

Some time later, I knew you'd get the odd smile, a bit of cooing and an occasional 'mama' or 'dada'. But after that, I admit to being a bit hazy until the bit where they go trotting off to the Infants' class, tripping over their uniform ('room to grow') and lugging a satchel that is bigger than they are.

I obviously wasn't listening when people filled in the gaps – therefore I had no clue as to the sheer speed at which small children change from burbling bairns to rampaging rugrats. Nor quite how quickly they can move when they have a mind to and how I would come to spend my days stooping to remove my darling daughter from cupboards, fireplaces and the numerous other places where she likes to get herself stuck. Note to self – must call osteopath.

How fast we have reached the point where we have to give dolly her tea before we eat our own, where we must wash all the teddies' faces before getting ourselves clean (with a now rather fluffy flannel). Had I known that the gourmet treats I had in store would consist solely of a plastic egg fed lovingly to me on a plastic spatula, I'd have paid more attention to stocking the freezer.

I have tried to think back to when I was that age – though frankly it was so long ago that my memories have apparently been filed on floppy disk, Betamax or some other now-obsolete format. I have hazy recollections of pounds, shillings and pence and, a little later, of cutting my panda's 'fingernails' and being aghast when all the stuffing fell out of his arms. I can muster a vague recall of Haliborange tablets every morning and aspirations of legs growing long enough to be allowed to ride the next-door neighbour's Chopper … though that's about it.

But they do say that the apple doesn't fall far from the tree, so perhaps it should have come as no great shock to learn that my daughter likes a natter. Fourteen months she may be, but just like her mother (and her paternal great-grandmother before her, a woman who single-handedly kept BT in business in the years between 1976 and the early part of the 21st century), she believes it's good to talk. Life these days comes with commentary:

Get dressed:
'Gocks!' (aka socks – though no, in our house they are now most definitely 'gocks'); 'top … knick knicks … '

Put on jewellery (rare):
'Necklet – ooh' (tug, break, etc.).

Visit friend's newborn son:
'Baby. Arry. Ahhhhhhhhhh. Cuggle.'

Proffer breadstick:
'Oooh – snack.'

Drop cup:
'Uh-oh. Wet.'

Pop to supermarket:
'App-le, nec-rine' (fruit aisle). 'Arry, Arry … ' (pictures of babies – on nappy packets or just about anywhere else).

And so it continues. Every day more words appear from nowhere and each time this little voice says something new my heart swells with pride. But it's dangerous territory.

Yesterday she gained unauthorised access to our bedroom and was discovered, guilty faced, clutching contraband in each fist.

'What's in your hand?' Little fingers open to reveal treasure. 'Keys, Mummy.' 'And what's in your other hand?' The other set of fingers unfurl. 'Car key.'

Her great escape may be thwarted – but I realise how easily I am swayed by her grasp of language – admonishment displaced by pride and discipline down the toilet. Must do better.

Her powers of observation grow daily and, with them, her idiosyncrasies. I guess I will never know why the word 'kiwi' can only be said in a voice that sounds like Donald Duck, nor why lions always roar in the quietest whisper. Maybe I am more concerned about the day she will point to my midriff and say 'spare tyre' instead of 'tum tum'. It can only be a matter of time.

Alas, however, my plans to show off my daughter's prowess have not always come to fruition. At a family gathering, I was proud as punch as she identified the guests by name:

Who's this? (pointing to me)   'Mummy'

Who's this? (pointing to husband)   'Daddy'

Who's this? (pointing to Mum)   'Gam-ma'

Who's this? (pointing to nephew)   'Poo poo'
(followed by uproarious laughter)

Then, admiring the stained-glass window on the stairs, 'Can you show Auntie how you can say "window", darling?'

'Turkey.'

Her latest trick is to follow any guest who decides to use the facilities, shouting, 'Wee wee, wee wee,' at the top of her voice. It seems that the Victorians may have had a point when they said that children should be seen and not heard.

Before we run into any more 'situations', I decide it might be time to move our focus away from verbal development and put our efforts into movement instead.

Sure, the child has got crawling and climbing down to a fine art but she has hitherto not so much as taken a step. Unlike her friends – *all* her friends – she has resolutely rejected every offer of instruction and gone out of her way to ignore the walker at all costs.

Of course, actions may speak louder than words – but apparently not in her book. Her language continues to improve daily in leaps and bounds – yet her defiant determination to travel in a horizontal, rather than vertical stance is such that I've begun to wonder whether she's gone all 'Animal Farm' on me. 'Four legs good, two legs bad', and all that.

And then, out of the blue, everything changes. 'Walk,' she says, clambering to her feet. And walk she does – right around the room, capping her performance off with a celebratory jig and a spot of jumping up and down. A few small steps for girl perhaps – but one giant leap for girlkind.

Suddenly, there is no stopping her. She runs everywhere at a pace – waving her arms about her head to indicate to all around her that, 'No assistance will be needed, thank you, even if you are thinking of trying to hold my hand to stop me running round in circles, rather than heading for home or throwing myself down the big girls' slide while my mother has yet another panic attack.'

I may be gaining grey hairs at the rate of knots, but I'm still as proud as Punch, Judy and probably the dodgy wooden crocodile too.

Our first proper family break – and while I know my memory is not what it once was, I could have sworn that when Cliff Richard crooned that he was going on a summer holiday he mentioned something about the sun shining brightly and the sky being blue. I am also pretty sure that his luggage didn't include wellies, waterproofs and hot-water bottles; yet as I pack for our trip to Norfolk you'd be hard pressed to tell if it is July or December from the contents of our cases.

Had we headed for the Continent, I'm sure we'd have been assured of sun aplenty. But when we considered the list of things we wanted to take with us and calculated what it would cost us in excess baggage, we realised that the choice was simple: remortgage or stay close to home.

It is probably for the best in any case, as the baby does not believe in travelling light. Whether she is a reincarnated war child I guess I will never know, but her insistence on stockpiling anything and everything she sees can surely have no other explanation.

How such small hands can hold so many things at once is surely a miracle of medical science, for she is never to be seen without at least seven assorted items clutched tightly to her bosom at any time during waking hours. A typical selection might include Bear (always Bear), a plastic teaspoon, a small pot, her 'handbag', a nasty-looking and distinctly seen-better-days breadstick, a now rather battered thank-you card and her old friend, the grey rubber doorstop. As she tries to add ever more miscellany to her haul, I am reminded of that bit in *The Generation Game*, where the winner accumulates an equally diverse variety of prizes (only in this case we don't get to take home a shiny new deep-fat fryer, a fondue set or an electric blanket).

Still, at least now that she is walking she is able to cart around her spoils without impeding her progress, whereas in the days of crawling it was a more complicated procedure altogether. Clank – the sound of a fistful of plastic ephemera hitting the wooden floor. Clunk. That's a brick. Hey ho – may have played havoc with my polished finish, but at least you could always hear her coming.

And so it is that laden with cases and clutter and an array of plastic accessories, we chug out of our driveway and head east, the car grumbling like a beast of burden and me WAP-ping the five-day forecast every 15 minutes. Heavy rain. No – it's changed to thundery showers. No – heavy rain it is …

To make matters worse, the purchase of a new(ish) car has done something strange to my husband, turning him from a perfectly normal bloke into a stranger whose only topics of conversation are body-coloured bumpers, interior trim and miles per gallon. I am half expecting him to make an unscheduled turn-off in search of driving gloves or a selection of nylon socks to go with his sandals. The baby and I focus on rousing choruses of 'The Wheels on the Bus' by way of distraction.

It seems de rigueur to stop off at a Little Chef for lunch – and after the obligatory egg on toast, we all feel much brighter. The baby finally achieves her ambition of getting a whole pot of grapes into her mouth in one go, although every time she moves her jaw to chew, strangers at neighbouring tables are peppered with a hail of green bullets. We beat a hasty retreat.

Despite the forecasts, fortune smiles upon us. The sun does shine brightly and we build sandcastles on the beach, bottle-feed lambs and make friends with the horses at the end of the garden. Plus, the baby's newfound walking prowess enables her to spend hour after happy hour wobbling up and down the rented cottage's gravel drive-way and revelling in the unfamiliar crunch beneath her feet.

Proper old-fashioned fun with lashings of ginger beer – it could almost be an Enid Blyton tale, just minus the mysterious strangers and Timmy the dog.

The trip is almost perfect – but for the fact that the baby takes agin the travel cot, forgoing her usual 7.30am start for daily protest at the crack of dawn.

We return home exhausted; in fact, in need of a holiday.

With the walking now down to a fine art, the child needs shoes – and fast.

This should not be an issue, at least on paper. After all, women, I am told, love to buy shoes. But it seems that there is something wrong with my genetic make-up: I do not love to buy shoes. I do not even remotely like to buy shoes. And now that I have to buy them for the baby too, my pleasure in this task has dissipated still further.

To be fair, contrary to footwear forays in the past, I had actually been looking forward to this particular one. The very first pair? A special day. Forget the sandals, the lightweight canvas of summer. Proper shoes. And a proper milestone.

We set out on our expedition to a shoe shop of repute. Aah, one of the seminal moments of mother-hood, I think, blinking back a tear or two of emotion as I pick out teeny, dainty pink slippers fit for any princess.

But then I glance across at my tomboy of a child, who is looking distinctly unregal as she plays football with a pair of discarded pop socks, and I return them to the shelf with a sigh.

I guess they wouldn't have fitted her in any case. Our budding David Beckham is somewhat large of foot. Which is probably why we call her flipper girl.

The assistant suggests ankle boots and brings out a pair of sturdy clodhoppers, which would have made even Tinkerbell look like a navvy. The shoes I like are too narrow. My second choice out of stock. We leave empty-handed.

Shop two. This time on a trip up North, so Grandma gets to come too, chuffed to bits to be part of the small girl's big day. The ones we want? Not available. We try some more.

'Can you walk in them?' asks the assistant a little too loudly, in the hope that volume might make up for any lack of vocabulary on the baby's part.

'Yes, walking,' says the child in an impressively withering tone, as she parades up and down the shop. 'And marching. And stomping. And jumping … ' They do not fit.

Shop three. A whole new range on offer. None, alas, to our taste. We pick out the pair we dislike the least. 'That'll be 80 pounds,' says the assistant.

Exit, pursued by a bear.

Shop four. And hurrah – the ones I had admired on another child of our acquaintance are in stock. The shoes that are neither fluorescent, nor sequinned, nor available only in narrow fittings. Better still, they do not necessitate a second mortgage. Eureka. Except … 'She has a very high instep,' says the assistant. 'No, sorry, these just aren't going to go on.'

Shop five. Discussions about high insteps. Advice that a T-bar shoe is the way forward. At last – progress.

But (of course there is a but …) the only pair available in her size is white patent. Judging by the way the child is hanging upside down off the bench by her toes ('swinging, Mummy – like a monkey') they will last precisely 15 seconds.

By now, I am having recurring dreams starring Prince Charming and a job lot of glass slippers that are too big, too small, too tight, too loose.

I'm sure that it was nowhere near this tricky when I was a girl – though possibly because choice hadn't yet been invented. Winter? Off to Clarks for a nice pair of sturdy lace-ups. Summer? A charming sandal available in brown or … oh, just brown. I guess that times have changed.

Fortunately, diligent research provides me with a list of further footwear emporia to try.

And so we set off for shop six. The baby looks a slightly odd shade of green en route, but I put this down to an understandable aversion to shoe shopping that is clearly contagious among those living in close confinement.

I find a parking space (slightly more taxing than finding a needle in an extremely large haystack), then out comes the buggy, in goes the child and … bleurgh. Buggy, baby, pavement dripping. I will spare you the graphic detail of the day of projectile puking that ensues, but suffice to say – no new shoes.

It may be worth me adding at this point that there are many careers that would really not have been for me, but chief among them is probably being a doctor, nurse or indeed anything else that involves dealing with bodily fluids on a professional basis. Despite the fact that I hail from a medical family, I am possibly the most squeamish person in Europe.

It is immensely good fortune that, other than her penchant for posseting, the child has not really put this failing of mine to the test for the best part of a year and a half. But when the moment finally arrives, I am truly found lacking.

One might summarise the scene thus:

One deserted street. One toddler (small, shoeless). One cascade of vomit (large, pungent). One inept mother.

The poor child has no idea what is happening and starts to weep and ask for cuddles. What I want to do is a) run away, b) cry and c) say, 'Don't be ridiculous, you are covered in steaming and stinking puke and I am not going anywhere near you.'

What I actually do is strip her down to her only-slightly-vomity vest, hyperventilate and retch a lot and make cuddly loving sort of noises while holding her as far away from myself as I possibly can and praying for a knight on a white charger to appear from nowhere with a bottle of Dettox, a washing machine and a fast ticket outta here.

I am a bad person.

The child falls asleep in the car seat and I bundle the sopping, stinking clothes and buggy into the boot, cursing the fact that it is unseasonably warm and that by the time we get home, therefore, the overpowering stench will have baked its way indelibly into everything in its path.

A load more vomit ensues, and each time I try to console from as great a distance as possible. Fortunately, the child is a very good patient. Whether this is down to her nature or the fact that she can sense my incompetence I do not know, but I suspect it is in large part due to the fact that she figures that a little charm might win her not only brownie points, but possibly extra medication to boot.

'Just a little tiny bit more pink medicine,' she entreats, looking cutely clammy. 'Or white medicine? Little bit of white medicine. I not very well.'

(The child's penchant for pharmaceutical potions is nothing new. 'I need powders,' she demands when her teeth are playing up, gums raw and saliva overload transferring itself to any nearby piece of clothing, bedding or other sundries. 'Little bit of powders. One more powders. Ooh – I need pink powders.'

But I have read those stories about Hollywood stars addicted to over-the-counter pain medication and, while Calpol has never actually been mentioned by name, I figure I'd better tread carefully nonetheless.)

Incidentally – the next time the baby vomits (always when her father is out – is she doing this on purpose?) I am infinitely braver. I wrap her in a towel and sit her on the floor while I deal with the sheets and tell her I just need to clear up the sick.

'Sick,' she says thoughtfully. 'Seven eight nine ten? Clever girl.'

The wee one has recovered and we drag ourselves forlornly back to the footwear fiasco. Exhausted by our efforts, by the time we make it to shop seven, both the baby and I are considering emigrating to a Pacific island where we can go barefoot forever more.

But – no, not a mirage – there they are. The perfect shoes. T-bar? Check. Absence of sequins? Check. Sensible colour? Check.

I hold my breath as the assistant slides them on to the baby's feet …

A perfect fit.

Yes, I know, in another six weeks' time we'll have to go through the whole thing again, but for now they're just the job. So it seems that Cinderella shall go to the ball after all.

*

After the vicissitudes of shoe shopping (and the toll taken thereof) it does cross my mind once again that perhaps if I was younger I would be better equipped to deal with the rigours of running around after a little one. And everyone of my own age that I ask about motherhood in 'mid-life' (apparently the polite way to say 'middle age') says the same – that they are permanently knackered and have far less energy than they did in their 20s.

True exhaustion is something that crops up in conversation with my mummy mates of any age. But when I ask one buddy (aged 31) what else she chats about on a night out with her friends she tells me: 'Oh, you know, the usual: fashion, films, music, gigs we've got tickets for … stuff everyone talks about really.'

I am sure that there are older mums who, despite their age, are also cool and trendy and go to concerts, but clearly I don't mix with any of them. I think back to my last night out with the girls (can you still use the word 'girls' when we are all the wrong side of 40?) and realise that what we discussed was as follows:

1) Prolapses.
2) Professional oven-cleaning services (indeed I admit I got way too excited at the idea of someone coming to my house and doing it for me – should really have apologised to fellow diners)

3) Colonic irrigation (no thanks).
4) M & S's new range of 'suck-you-in' pants (ooh – perhaps that counts as fashion?).

But another topic has begun to rear its head – a more difficult one, which seems to be inveigling its way into conversations with friends of all ages: baby number two.

One of the younger mums is already pregnant again. Another has recently given birth and a third is currently the size of a small village and due any minute. They talk about how they want to get their families out of the way now, so that by the time they're 50 the kids will have flown the nest and they will be free to hitchhike around India and turn the empty bedrooms into fitness suites and home offices and such like.

Other friends, also with time on their side, are in no rush, and decide to space things out a bit and continue their climb up the career ladder.

But for us older mums, it's not so simple …

A dear friend, a doctor who is never one to mince his words, asks when I'm going to go for number two:

'I'm not. I'm too old,' I tell him.

'Don't be silly, what are you – 40, 41?'

'44.'

'Oh yes, you really are too old, aren't you?'

As it happens, I know several women who have given

birth in their mid-, even late 40s without any problems at all. But there are many, many reasons why I feel I ought to stick at one: I don't want to push my luck. I am not sure I could cope with the emotional stress and worries of a second geriatric pregnancy. I have never been very good at peeing into pots with any kind of accuracy and really cannot face going through the whole aiming-and-missing thing again on a regular basis, not least in a toilet that is plastered with signs about what you can and can't flush in order to avoid leakage into the wards situated beneath.

Oh, I have thought long (so long) and hard about having a second child, but in the end have decided, with regret, not to give it a go.

My head knows that for me, this is the right decision. My heart is having trouble keeping up. 'Look at that cute little newborn,' it screams every time we pass a pram in the street. 'Remember how snuggly and sweet they are?' And every time we go shopping it just needs to be within a hundred yards of a babywear department to deafen me with taunts of, 'Look at these adorable teeny tiny clothes. You know you want them. You do … '

And oh, I do. I do, I do, I do.

To make matters harder, it seems that almost every day yet another friend announces the impending arrival of number two, number three … But while I am thrilled for them – and truly, I am – I admit that there is also a tinge of jealousy over the fact that they are the proud possessors of 30-something ovaries and whippersnapper wombs.

I feel more blessed than I will ever be able to articulate to have my darling daughter – yet it breaks my heart not to do all this again (especially as next time round I might actually have a clue as to what I was doing). How I would love to feel those kicks and flutters deep within me just one more time, touch the swell of my stomach and know there is a whole new life growing inside. But deep down, I know it's not to be.

I am not alone in feeling this way though, and it is a comfort to know that many older mums have also struggled long and hard over the do we/don't we question. Seems there's nothing like a bit of broody bonhomie.

One friend says, 'If I go for another, I'll be 43 plus – and the experience of having an amnio while feeling the child moving inside me is just not something I can put myself through again. I do feel sad about it though – and if I was younger, I would have more children without question.'

Even those who do decide to give it a go are only too aware of the overwhelming pressure to get in there before the biological clock runs out of tock:

'I would definitely prefer not to have to do it right now and would like to take longer over trying for number two, but I don't have the time. But then I also worry about having two very young children so close together and the energy needed at my age.'

Every mum I have ever met has good days and bad days – times when they want to shout to the world that motherhood is the greatest thing in the universe, and times when they want to hide under the duvet with a family pack of Flakes and their hands firmly clamped over their ears (which, now I think about it, could present an interesting logistical challenge when it comes to actually consuming the aforementioned chocolate – and that's before you even start to consider what it would do to the bedclothes).

But my own experience – and that of my friends – has shown that there are actually many plusses to being a slightly more mature mum. As one says:

'I am fairly (usually? occasionally?) calm and relaxed and certainly more self-assured than I would have been a decade ago; I appreciate how lucky I am having so nearly missed out on my dream. Plus, my daughter will get to watch cool programmes such as *Mr Benn* and *Bagpuss*.'

And I know that I too appreciate being a mum in a way I probably wouldn't have at 30. I revel in those moments of exquisite happiness and don't worry about what I might be missing out on – as I may well have done had I been younger.

"Ah – but the downside,' says Sam, who is something of a sage in such matters having had three kids in her 20s, then a fourth in her 40s, 'is that it costs a bloody fortune on upkeep. I will always be dyeing my hair because I categorically refuse to be a grey-haired mum at the primary-school gates.'

And she has a point.

I look around at my counterparts, at the young ones and at those who are old, but frankly in way better nick than I am, and I realise that a little sprucing up may be long overdue.

Just how long overdue is brought home to me by my husband when I am serving up a supper of spag bol and manage to drop both the pasta on the floor and the sauce all over the cooker.

'Are you menopausal or something?' he asks, although when he notices I have a carving knife in my hand (for the garlic bread, I hasten to add) he backtracks with, 'I mean premenstrual.'

But the damage is done.

'So you're saying that even you think of me as middle aged?' I storm, dropping his dinner into the bin and rushing off to examine my hairline in the mirror.

I realise that I do not want my husband to see me as

an aged crone, nor am I able to bear the thought of my daughter enduring endless playground taunts about how I'm old enough to be her granny. And so I am left with no alternative but to start putting some decent effort into becoming a yummy mummy.

But there's a lot to do, and it's going to be an uphill battle.

Years of tonsorial tussles with dryers, straighteners, crimpers (yes, yes, it was the '80s) have proved that unless there is substantial professional or chemical involvement, my hair never quite looks neat. This is borne out one day at nursery pick-up:

Grandmother (to the small boy in her arms who is pointing at me and shouting, 'Mama, mama'): No, darling, that's not your mummy. Although your mummy does have a similar hairstyle.

Me (to grandmother): I hope it's not as messy as mine, ha ha ha …

Grandmother (to me): Well sometimes it is, but most of the time hers is beautiful.

I take to wearing a hood.

As it happens, my hair has actually been a source of great angst since way back when – with me insisting that the tight curls be allowed to grow until they got long enough to afford me the delights of the ponytails and plaits that my primary-school comrades were all able to enjoy, nay flaunt, with such gay abandon … and my mother refusing and taking me to have it shorn on a regular basis, thus ensuring a pudding bowl of frizz that has haunted me to this day. (Although, in her defence, when I was – finally – old enough to fight off the scissors, it was a long and painful process to get my hair to a point where it might be styled in any way whatsoever.)

Indeed, when I look back at photos of my early teenage years it is often impossible to discern whether or not I am wearing a dark brown motorcycle helmet. And even when it finally did grow long, I was not yet out of the woods. During a recent clearout I came across a cutting I had kept from a 1990 edition of the *Radio Times* featuring me, Terry Wogan and the rest of our chat-show production team. I showed it to my husband who looked at me aghast and asked how on earth I had got away with sporting a small furry animal on top of my head while at work (which was surely a contravention of health and safety laws even then).

I have fantasised that any child of mine will be blessed with poker-straight hair, thus to spare her many years of tress-related trauma and many miserable hours of agonising knot removal but alas, on this front it is already clear that my prayers have gone unheard. As soon as she is able to articulate her desires, the child asks piteously for hair adornments as worn by all of her friends. I do relent and buy her a clip, but once it is in place it is invisible to the naked eye (and indeed it takes many moments of frantic foraging to relocate it among the rampaging curls).

The poor child has also inherited her parents' pallor, meaning that in years to come I will have to sit her down for that difficult conversation about the advent of summer and share with her all that I was forced to learn about the art of fake tan (a lesson stemming from an unfortunate episode involving the glare from the white, white legs that I foolishly dared to bare on the first warm day of the season and the resultant traffic incident caused by dazzled and traumatised drivers on the local high road).

Not that covering up always makes things any better. While many other mothers manage to make chain-store bargains look like haute couture, with me the opposite is true and even the smartest of outfits somehow falls slightly askew the moment I put it on.

It would no more occur to me to put on lipstick of a morning than it would to fly to the moon. I have never been able to walk in high heels. Perhaps I am a hopeless case … not least because I do not have a four-wheel drive in which to negotiate the rough terrain of the Brent

Cross car park. And, come to that, I also loathe shopping with a passion.

Worse still – I fear my dear child is truly her mother's daughter. As a newborn, while all the other little girls cooed daintily in their immaculate outfits, mine was already laughing like Sid James and was always missing a sock.

Now, as her contemporaries dress up as fairies and trip delicately around the room, my girl charges at me like a bull in a china shop, requesting yet another game of football.

Ah well. Perhaps I should simply follow her lead and embrace the people we are, not what we, or others, think we ought to be.

So bye bye notions of yummy mummyhood. I bid you farewell as I head off for a good old kick around. My mascara will remain unused, my blusher pristine in its unopened box, the nail bar a place of mystery.

Instead, you'll find us jumping in puddles, or making mud pies down the park with our mad hair blowing in the wind. And that's just the way we like it.

The days whizz past and the child's eccentricities become ever more apparent and, correspondingly, my devotion to this madcap moppet grows ever deeper.

I do not chastise her for refusing to go to sleep, crying piteously because she wants to hold a magic wand (why? I have no idea). As I am about to go out for dinner, I tell her that if she does go to sleep then we shall play with a magic wand in the morning. (This despite the fact that we do not have a magic wand – and thus I am up until the early hours, doing my level best with a drumstick and a roll of Bacofoil and hoping I'll get away with it.)

Nor can I get annoyed in the dead of night when she wakes me calling that she 'must have a recipe; for garlic bread'.

Instead, I revel in the things that seemed so boring before she came along, loving the fact that when I take her to the supermarket she insists on waving to all the (very dead) fish, blowing kisses to the 'yummy yummy' olives and yelling, 'Let's dunk,' as we pass the biscuit aisle.

It is hard to believe that a year and a half has already flown by. A year and a half in which I have had more fun than I could ever have imagined. A year and a half in which it would be fair to say that we have established that motherhood is one steep learning curve. (Latest lesson: elderly relative seating toddler on upholstered armchair and presenting it with a cream cheese bridge roll is not a good idea – essentially the equivalent of handing it a pot of white emulsion, a brush and free rein with your soft furnishings.)

But given this and countless other examples – which, be thankful, I shall spare you – I do wonder how it is that I continue to be surprised when I discover yet another new thing I never realised I needed to know.

Let us observe a case in point.

For the majority of my 40-something years a park has been – well, a park. Nice, green space. A few dogs. The odd tree. A swing or two. In my younger days, I would have been delighted by a tennis court. Now a café will do me just fine. But, basically, nothing too far off the standard dictionary definition.

These days, however, it's not so simple. A park is not a park. Just as the wolf donned a frilly bonnet and pretended to be sweet rosy-cheeked grandmamma, so this green patch of land has hoodwinked me into believing it is an innocent play space, not a hotbed of social complexities.

Oh why did no one warn me about Park Etiquette?

My ignorance has meant I have been forced to learn the hard way that it is *never* okay to tell someone else's child to get off the slide, even if they are standing on your own offspring's ears.

Nor must you raise an eyebrow when someone tells you their son is named after a football stadium (Stamford – as in Bridge).

Moreover, it is bad form to laugh at a poor bald baby

done up in a big flowery hair bow, even if she does look like an Easter egg.

There really ought to be a degree course in Playground Politics. At least then you would be equipped with the knowledge that certain mothers are 'in the queue' for the swings before they have even left home. And woe betide you if you try to make a case for those who are actually standing there in line.

Also, you would know never to stare at someone who looks barely out of nappies themselves, asking yourself – is that the baby's mother or their sister? That way you are fully justified in feeling affronted when you sense someone's gaze upon your good self, wondering – is that the kid's mother or her grandmother?

And it has become clear that I'm not the only member of our family who has a lot to learn.

On a recent trip, we strolled across the grass and the baby took a shine to a canoodling couple in the distance. Before I could explain that when it comes to romantic trysts, three is most definitely a crowd, she had rushed off and hauled herself up on to the bench beside them, leaning back with a satisfied sigh.

'Chair. Big girl,' she told the couple proudly.

Then, taking their smiles as encouragement, she lifted her top. 'Tummy,' she said, solemnly pointing to her midriff. 'Button' – one finger in her navel.

I finally caught up with her as she was regaling them with descriptions of her shoes and socks. They were terribly nice about it and accepted my apologies most graciously – but they did run for the hills as quickly as courtesy allowed.

It is possibly best to gloss over the visit to another local play space, when the baby ambled past a group of picnickers and, using sleight of hand that would have put any Dickensian pickpocket to shame, reappeared at my side clutching a fish finger dripping in ketchup.

And there's another thing – contrition is all very well, but it's not that simple to return a seafood snack when it's covered in teeth marks ...

But as autumn draws to a close and the chill winds and rains arrive in force, at least we are granted respite, some time to learn to mend our ways.

I will try to curb my daughter's kleptomania and teach her that not every Labrador in London belongs to her cousins – therefore it is not necessary for her to throw herself at each and every dog we see shouting, 'Bagel! Woof! Waggy waggy.'

And as for me? I shall draw the curtains and curl up on the sofa with a copy of *Debrett's*, and perhaps by the time spring rolls around I shall know my stuff.

CHAPTER 8

18–24 MONTHS

Once upon a time there were three bears. Not, as the story would have it, a mummy bear, a daddy bear and a baby bear, but three identical bears. And they lived, not in a cottage in the woods, but in a cot or a wardrobe, depending on which point of the rotational cycle they were at.

When one bear was beginning to look a little past his prime, he would be whisked off to rehab and replaced, in the dead of night when small people were snoring, by another bear – slightly fresher, perhaps, but in all other ways indistinguishable from his cohort.

The happy ending to this story is entirely dependent upon this cycle of strict rotation, ensuring that no bear remains pristine and smelling of 'new', and all become interchangeably bedraggled at the earliest opportunity.

There is, perhaps, no finer illustration than this of the benefits of being an older mother. You inherit the wisdom and experience of all the friends who've been there before you and sometimes, just sometimes, you really learn from their mistakes (in this case, never to underestimate what the loss of an offspring's favourite toy can do to your nerves and your sleep patterns).

It is thanks to such insight that a small girl of my acquaintance is never parted from her beloved friend, even when unforeseen and unfortunate incidents occur – although I am sure there will soon come a time when she will understand that her parents' vomit-removing capacities are duplicitous rather than superhuman.

Perhaps this is the time to confess that this popular ursine fable is not the only tale to have been tinkered with in our household.

Take the old woman who lived in a shoe. I really don't want to paint my daughter a picture of scores of children being whipped soundly before turning in for the night … So our version has the over-fertile crone reading them a story before they trot off to bed. Still without any bread – after all, there is tampering and there is tampering. Dr Atkins would be proud.

Looking at them anew, this time from an adult perspective, it becomes clear that the majority of nursery rhymes are not terribly child friendly. To say the least.

Oranges and Lemons? Decapitation. London Bridge? Beyond repair. Three Blind Mice? Dismembered. And so it goes on.

These days, it seems that every time I open our book of traditional rhymes and ditties I find myself getting a little maudlin. It may, of course, be my hormones, but that doesn't stop me shedding a tear for all those poor people who fall down dead from the plague in Ring O Roses.

Then there's the misfortune befalling the innocent folk of Gloucester, left without any medical cover, all because Dr Foster doesn't have the perspicacity to look where he's going.

And what about that poor maid, left to do all the chores, while her fat-cat employers count their cash and stuff themselves silly on sweet treats? And all she gets by way of thanks is the loss of her nose. Although I can't say I really blame any blackbird that has the fortitude to make it through the pie fiasco unscathed for being just a little bit narky.

Who'd have thought that reading children's stories could be such a minefield? Last night I spent half an hour comforting a weeping toddler girl who had taken a singsong session too much to heart.

'Poor Humpty Dumpty,' she sobbed. 'Fell down banged 'is 'ead. Broken.'

And 'Chicken Licken' has had to be banished forever more after my traumatised child woke up protesting, 'But I don't want to go and tell the king that the sky is falling in. I want to watch *Peppa Pig*.'

But that's not to say that there are no tales more suited to my sensibilities: as it happens I am in total accordance with mummy cat's position of no pie, for if the little kittens have lost their mittens they surely need to learn that carelessness has consequences?

However, the constant explanations vis-à-vis the welfare of folk involved in the more mawkish tales is taking its toll on one frazzled mummy – so for the sake of all our nerves, perhaps we'll be sticking exclusively with 'Twinkle Twinkle' for a while.

And so here we find ourselves, a little older, a little greyer and usually to be heard singing about diamonds in the sky (me); and a little older, considerably taller and usually to be found holding a 'handbag' containing a hair clip, a pair of sunglasses, a slice of wooden birthday cake, a rubber ice-cube tray and an empty raisin box (her).

I would like to think that – nursery-rhyme censorship apart – since becoming a mother I have learned a great deal. Perhaps you will allow me to demonstrate this by sharing with you the most salient points:

1) Do not expect a sensible answer to a sensible question

For example:

Q 'Darling, why are you lying in the wet and dirty mud in the middle of the park?'

A 'I am sleeping.'

Q 'Okay. And may I ask why you are sleeping?'

A 'I am dreaming.'

2) Do not ask rhetorical questions

My 'And what shall we wear today?' (which is somewhat academic, given I already have her jeans and top in my hand) is met by a decisive, 'Spotty jim jams, two pink plates and an umbrella.'

3) 'W' is the most overused letter of the alphabet

I had not realised until now that 'wingers' are not Ryan Giggs, Theo Walcott et al., but the digits on the ends of one's hands. Likewise, in the morning I take a 'wower' and, correspondingly, our favourite vegetable is 'cauli-wower'. And, as certain sibilant sounds are also proving tricky to master, I would agree with Elton John that yes, 'wo-wee' really does seem to be the hardest word.

4) Procrastination may be the thief of time – but no one told the baby

Nineteen months old and already her answer to everything is, 'In a minute' or, 'Hang on'.

5) Mummy does not always have the answer

A treat for breakfast. 'Do you know what it is, darling? It's a crumpet.'

'Crumpet. Ooooh.' Cups hands to mouth. 'Toot toot toot.' (How exactly does one explain the difference between a crumpet and a trumpet to a baby?)

6) There is always an excuse

The child is walking around the house, throwing her arms about dramatically, shouting, 'Oh god, the mess.'

And I thought it was quite tidy.

But that's before I discover what she has done to her room: all the wipes out of the packet ('I needed to wipe all the toys' bottoms'). And all the clothes on the floor ('because they are pretty').

7) Babies lack sophistication

For example, my daughter does not appreciate my *MasterChef* obsession, and rejects the quenelles of fish finger with a pea fricassée and sweetcorn foam asking for a 'wamwich' instead.

8) Two steps forward, one step back

Just when you think you have got somewhere, you discover that actually, you haven't got anywhere at all. Illustrated by a recent conversation that ended thus:

'So – what does a dog do with his tail?'

'Wag.'

'And what does a dog say?'

'Hello.'

'And what does a dog eat?'

'Carrots.'

'No, darling. A doggy eats a bone. Bone. So what does a rabbit eat?'

'Carrots.'

'And what do you eat?'

'A bone … '

9) You are never too young to fall in love

There are many objects of my daughter's affections. At bedtime we go through an ever-increasing list of them to establish that yes, baby Harry, Abi, Zoe … Meelia … the toy caterpillar … Peter Rabbit … the robin on the tissue box (and so on) are also drinking their milk like good boys/girls/fictitious animals.

But now there is a new love, someone she talks about day and night. Like a teenage girl outside the

X Factor house, she will do anything to catch even a fleeting glimpse of her hero, peering over my shoulder to scour every corner of the Friday playgroup in case he might be there.

When she spots him there is no containing her excitement. 'Hello, Rabbi,' she yells at the top of her voice. 'Waving at Rabbi, winking at Rabbi, blowing kiss to Rabbi.'

Her enthusiasm is not limited to his presence. At home the crayons come out and, 'Draw Rabbi,' she commands. 'One more Rabbi.'

While I am certainly an admirer of said rabbi, I am hoping that for the baby this will be a fleeting first love and thus we can avoid 'the conversation'.

For I still remember the bitter taste of misery at age two, when my parents gently explained to me that I wouldn't actually be able to marry my Uncle Charlie because he was already married (not to mention my uncle – and 30 years my senior; I guess there's only so much a heartbroken toddler can take in at one time.)

10) You can kid yourself – but you can't kid a kid …

Yes, I'm old, but the thing is that I forget that I am old most of the time. Sure, it's a bit of a shock to see myself in a photograph or a mirror, but even if I choose to keep my eyes tightly closed, it would appear that the days of deluding myself might be numbered.

My daughter sits upon my lap, gazing up at me adoringly, gently tracing the contours of my face with her fingers.

Aaah, I think, lump in throat. This is what it's all about. The inextricable bond between mother and daughter. And now she's showing that she understands it too.

Then, 'Mummy … ' she says. 'Lots of wrinkles.'

Short of spending my life savings on Botox, I don't suppose that there's much I can do on that front – but perhaps I should view this as my wake-up call. Previous efforts may have fallen by the wayside, but it is clear that action is needed – and fast.

And it appears that the child seems to think so too. Following her up the stairs, her awareness of my shortcomings becomes all too apparent. 'Come on, Mummy, nearly there, nearly there. Well done, Mummy!' she calls encouragingly. Not even two and already calling my fitness into question? It's alarming.

And so I've rejoined the gym, figuring that this may at least deal with some of the saggy and baggy bits, if nothing else.

It's been a while, what with babies and backs and stuff, and I'm more than a little nervous to have to squeeze into my sports kit and stagger off for a workout. Still, I am suffused with enthusiasm …

… until I actually get there, when it all starts to look a little bit like hard work. Even the bits where you can sit down turn out to be exhausting. And I must admit that I do question my motivation when I call it quits on the cross-trainer the moment I have burned off enough calories for a Cadbury Creme Egg (around 170, in case you are wondering).

'Do you think you have issues?' asks my husband, when I confess to him that I have found myself lying to the machines about my age and weight.

It would seem that the answer is yes.

'Stop worrying,' he says. 'You've just had a baby. It takes time.'

I am depressed to realise that, actually, the 'baby' is almost two, so perhaps this excuse is a little past its sell-by date. But the fact that he's trying so hard to cheer me up (including telling everyone that I am 'only thirty-fourteen' when my birthday rolls around) does at least make me love him all the more.

'I would never ever lie,' says a mate when I (foolishly) ask her opinion. 'What are you thinking of? Be out and proud.'

I have just assumed that everybody glosses over their age (and indeed weight) once they hit a certain point. But apparently, it's only me.

However, I do feel slightly better when one person (48 when she gave birth) admits, 'I've never actually lied, but I have withheld the information for a while before letting people know. Or just said, I was in my 40s when I had Lucy … '

Which seems fair enough to me – after all – omission is surely way down the scale of sin from fabrication? As a colleague once told me: 'I've never lied about my age – I simply avoid mentioning it, or have a moment of being hard of hearing if someone brings it up. Someone drew up a contact list for our toddler group. They wanted the mums' birthdays as well as the children's. All the other mums included their birth year (why?), but my pen handily ran out after I'd written just the date and the month. What luck … '

However, bar these (very) few comrades, everyone else I speak to seems to think that even implication is to be frowned upon and that out-and-out untruths are the equivalent of drowning poor defenceless little puppies or torturing kittens or some such.

Perhaps the problem is that I am going through a phase of feeling my age more than usual. This is partly due to the number of younger mummy mates discussing plans to go to Glastonbury (and making me conscious of the fact that where once I too would have enjoyed nothing more than a night under canvas, now the noise, lack of facilities and absence of an orthopaedic mattress would turn me into a very grumpy old woman indeed). And largely due to an unaccustomed lack of sleep.

The baby has more or less a full set of gnashers, achieved almost without bother, but now her molars are giving her gip. She is chewing, pooing, and dribbling relentlessly, and sometimes, in the dead of night, the pain becomes too much.

A friend, noting the toll that this has taken on both me and the nipper, suggests that whisky might be the way forward. And so I take a bottle to bed and when the cries start up at 3am, I take a good slug and instantly feel much better. I'm out like a light, leaving my husband on dentistry duty, and in the morning I can actually open my eyes without having to resort to a chisel.

'What great advice,' I tell my chum when we catch up later in the day. 'I didn't hear a thing.' But it turns out she had actually been advocating an old-fashioned remedy whereby the alcohol is intended for the *child* and rubbed on to the offending gums in order to dull the pain.

Ah.

*

It seems it's really not my week.

We are invited to a parent-and-child 'messy play' session at nursery. Figuring that we're going to get covered in paint, glue, glitter and the like, we don our oldest jeans and T-shirts and head off for an afternoon of sticking, scribbling and smearing.

Then, in come the other mothers. They are statuesque (even the ones who are heavily pregnant). They are elegantly dressed. They are wearing high heels. Their hair, neither in need of a wash nor scrunched roughly into ponytails, is all shiny and shampoo-adverty. Worst of all (as I mentally flick through my book of age-related excuses in order to have one at the ready), I note that not all of them are young.

I want to ask, 'Did you not think there was a clue in the word "messy"? Do you not realise that your designer clothes and your perfect manicures will never stand up to the rigours of poster paint and Play-Doh?'

But, in fact, although they seem to throw themselves into the proceedings with every bit as much gusto as I do, they also leave every bit as immaculately as they arrived. Naturally, the same cannot be said for me or for the child – who has green paint in her hair, blue on (and up) her nose and red glitter pretty much everywhere else.

The final blow (kick me when I'm down, Mrs Alpha mother – why don't you?) comes when a supermodel type (who is clearly thinking: I'll make an effort with the bag lady in the corner) says, 'I believe my Tabitha is in the same class as your little boy.'

I go home and hide under the duvet.

Adding insult to injury, winter has arrived with a vengeance and I've convinced myself that I am suffering from SAD.

It's cold, it's wet and pushing the buggy through the freezing rain and snow has lost its appeal.

It is true that in days gone by, I revelled in days like these, believing it was nature's way of telling me to turn up the heating, dial a pizza, curl up on the sofa with a good book and a duvet … and relax.

Even when the baby was small, inclement weather wasn't such an issue. After all, play mats are play mats, come rain or shine. Add a chorus of 'Baa Baa Black Sheep', a quick jiggle of Minnie Mouse and a couple of coochie-coos and, frankly, everyone's happy.

Now she's a toddler, it's not so simple. 'Out, out,' she implores, desperate to escape the confines of these four walls (and, no doubt, a mother who has parked herself under the anglepoise in a bid to recreate the sunlight of more clement climes).

But while I aim to please, I am less inclined to give in to pleas for 'park' and 'mud pies' in Arctic conditions, or when the rain falls in sheets and a force 10 gale howls around the house like a banshee.

It's a difficult age. (Hers … well, and mine.)

I pore over books of rainy-day activities, ruling out the many suggestions that involve paper clips (choking hazard), scissors (lethal) and string (having had to cut her free from the high chair once already).

I try the obvious and get out the crayons, but her constant requests to 'Draw Rabbi, Mummy, just one more,' do not allow for the free-flowing creativity I had envisaged.

Time for our failsafe – a spot of reading. She loves books, and between us we can now recite many children's classics by heart. But today *The Gruffalo*, *Each Peach Pear Plum* and all the others are out of favour – and only one book will do.

It's not that I have anything against our inherited copy of *My First Passover Board Book*, but I have discovered that there is a limit to how animated one can be when saying, 'Ooh, look, darling, Moses in a basket,' for the thirtieth time in one day.

She is oblivious to my antipathy.

Next, we try baking, her favourite activity, though I soon discover that babies are absolute rubbish when it comes to creaming butter and sugar to a mousse-like consistency.

I give her the task of mixing the dry ingredients instead and the small amount that stays in her bowl is added to mine before we do patting and rolling.

The kitchen looks like it's been hit by a blizzard and, as I transport our sweet treats to the oven, I have to tread carefully through clouds of icing sugar as well as heeding my daughter's counsel: 'Be careful. 'ot, 'ot. Burn your wingers.'

At bedtime, she proudly tells Daddy she made biscuits.

'And what did you put in the bowl?' he asks.

'Butter. Eggies. Sugar … '

'And?' he enquires.

'Cauli-wower.' It seems she has yet to grasp the concept of self-raising …

Another day, another deluge.

We want to run through the trees, jump in puddles, search for leaves. Instead, we are trapped once more as the flood waters rise outside and I ponder how long it would take to build an ark. Out of rice cakes.

By 10am, cabin fever has taken hold and I am overcome with exhaustion. I lie on the living-room floor, yawning loudly to illustrate my point.

'Mummy is very, very tired,' I tell her.

'Mummy really, really needs lots and lots of … ' I wait for her to say 'sleep', but no.

'Wine?' she suggests.

I think she has a point.

Now that she truly appears to have learned to call a spade a spade, it seems a very long time since my girl was a newborn. Of course, I appreciate that it stands to reason that just as I get older, so does she. But as I am in denial about my own ageing process and the fact that yet another birthday is now behind me, so I seem to forget that she is no longer a babe in arms, but a walking, talking toddler with something to say about everything.

One of her (many) current obsessions is hair:

'Mummy long hair.'
'Yes that's right, darling.'
'Me long hair.'
'Well, not really, but it's getting there, sweetie.'
'Daddy long hair.'

'Well Daddy doesn't really have any hair at all, darling – but probably best not to mention ... '

Another area of constant discussion is gender – and all that accompanies it:

'Boy have willies.'
'Yes, darling. That's right.'
'Daddy willie.'
'Well, yes.'
'Mummy willie.'
'No, darling – Mummy is a girl; girls do not have willies. What is Mummy?'
'A girl.'
'Well done – and what are you?'
'Hilarious.'

As it happens, the small fry's growing grasp of the differences between the sexes has provoked a new and strangely illuminating topic of conversation among the mums – namely what to call our offspring's 'bits'.

For the boys, it seems to be simple, with 99 per cent opting for 'willie' and just one per cent defiantly sticking to 'penis'. The 'winkles' and 'weenies' of my childhood – and yes, I realise that may sound slightly dodgy, but please remember that I was raised long ago in an era of innocence – appear to have faded with the mists of time.

The girls are another matter altogether. As someone who grew up using the utilitarian 'front bottom', I was both entranced and mystified by the fact that my best friend had a 'dig-ee-dog' (and 40 years later, I admit to being none the wiser as to how that came about).

I know of 'mutchies', 'putchies', 'peaches' and 'fairies'. One friend is insistent on 'vagina', while the rest shudder at its 'harshness' and plump for 'nunnie' or 'noo noo' instead. How my daughter ended up with a 'noodle' I am not entirely sure, though I am tempted to convince her to go with the one that my sister-in-law grew up with – after all, shouldn't every girl have a 'fanfare'?

The child says she has a tummy ache. I offer to rub it better and discover that she has been posting all the wooden animals from her Noah's ark down the front of her vest and there is a gorilla wedged between the top of her nappy and her navel.

We go to Tesco, where she informs the lady on the checkout – and the many gentlemen in the queue behind us – that 'my mummy wearing black knickers'.

(Mind you it could be worse. One friend – a devout Christian – was forced to seek an alternative place of worship after her four-year-old daughter informed the entire Sunday school, including the vicar, that 'Mummy's got a hairy bottom'. While a cousin's four-year-old son asked his mother if she shaved her moustache with Daddy. And a neighbour was forced to change jobs after her toddler daughter told her boss that his face was 'just like Grandad's'. Grandad has Bell's Palsy.)

But most of the time (or to be fair, pretty much all the time, bar when she divulges the details of my smalls to complete strangers), I revel in my girl's awareness of everything around her and love the way she tells it like it is.

For example, since the efficacy of the night-time nappy has been found lacking on a regular basis, her first greeting of the day has changed and now, instead of the more traditional, 'Morning, Mummy', I get either, 'Oh, sweetie pie, you're all wet' (on a bad day), or a cheery, 'Nice and dry' (on a good one).

As she speeds towards the terrible twos, I can't decide whether to bemoan the fact that her compliance is waning – or celebrate the fact she knows exactly what she wants. Yesterday's, 'I'm just going to make your supper, darling,' was met with a hopeful, 'Cous cous?' (Not a chance – a cheese sarnie.) And when I mention fruit for pudding:

'Nectarine?'

'No, darling – we don't have any nectarines.'

'Go to shop buy it.'

She had to make do with an apple.

My own childhood is so long ago that it is often hard to remember the voyage of discovery that I took into the wider world, though I do clearly recall weeping bitterly in the primary-school playground after a maths lesson when it became clear that 'tens and units' did not, after all, mean kitchen planning.

But perhaps the passage of time makes it all the more pleasurable to be exploring the world anew in my 40s. And I am learning lots.

My daughter assures me that leopards have 'spots', tigers have 'stripes' and lions? 'Have willies'. And we have a number of in-depth conversations about the fact that no, pitta bread and Peter Rabbit are not related.

In my daughter's version of the Old Testament the ark is manned by Iggle Piggle, while Noah drives a fire engine. And I am now led to understand, having listened closely to her singing herself to sleep, that I've been getting words wrong all over the place, and it's actually, 'Round and round the garden, like a teddy bear, one step, two steps, tickle you on the boo boos'.

Hey ho, at least it gives us gives us plenty to talk about and helps to take my mind off the depression that threatens to settle when I find myself filling out an application form and realise that there now seem to be five boxes above the one I am requested to tick to indicate my age – and only two below (one of which reads '65 and over').

On the days that I work, the girl goes to nursery – a fate which she appears to have adapted to rather quicker than her mother. There is a webcam ('See,' says my friend Jules, 'there's another advantage of starting later – when my kids were little there was nothing as fancy as that'), but whether it is actually a good thing or a bad thing I have yet to decide.

Yes, I love that I can see what she is up to and bear witness to her first independent steps into the big wide world. Yes, it is fantastic to get a real flavour of her day. But boy, is it a distraction, the temptation to stay tuned in with a family-sized bucket of popcorn being almost overwhelming, even in the face of yet another deadline.

Make long list of tasks to be crammed into the working day. Quick click to check that I did remember to put tights on her this morning. Lay the pages of the document

I have been sent to rewrite in front of me. Get slightly sidetracked by how she appears to be refusing to hold on to the barre in her 'ballet' lesson. Wrestle with synonyms and syntax. Another crafty peek to make sure she's eating all her lunch. And so on and so forth …

I start to feel like Bridget Jones's older sister:

Wednesday 9 December. Calories consumed – 3,000 (mainly popcorn). Weight gained: 9oz. New wrinkles – 4 (bad). Number of times tuned into nursery webcam – 628.

The festive season is approaching once again and I am spending every spare moment searching for a fairy costume for the nursery concert. My creativity is hampered by an uncharacteristic lack of sleep, although I know I should not be complaining about one bad night among the textbook seven till sevens.

I have yet to fathom the reason for the tears: the baby's explanations include, 'Peppa Pig is crying' (eh?), 'My Grobag is broken' (it isn't) and, 'My ankles need stroking'.

In the morning, she cannot eat her breakfast, 'Because the toast has a tummy ache'. So I pack up an industrial-size carton of breadsticks and we head for the local shopping centre in search of wings (we're still talking fairies here, rather than Claire Rayner, lest there be any confusion).

For the first time ever, mine is the child who will not stop screaming throughout the entire trip. I achieve nothing I set out to do and purchase only a large bottle of red before giving in and calling it a day. I try to calm her by pointing out the twinkly lights and then, at her request, singing 'Twinkle Twinkle' – 26 times without a break, until she falls asleep in the buggy. I am then unable to extricate my thumb and thus sit/stoop/slump at an awkward and ungainly angle for the next 40 minutes for fear of waking her. I gaze longingly at the wine and wish I didn't have to drive home.

A doctor's visit reveals raging infections in both her ears and that she had been screaming because she was in agony and because her mother was making her browse photo frames, instead of dosing her with Calpol and kissing it better (as requested).

And I was meant to know that how? Ah well, another lesson learned.

She has recovered and the time for the concert has arrived.

My husband and I arrive early to grab front-row seats for the grand performance. Even with half an hour to go, I am overwhelmed with the emotion of my baby's big day and my husband tries not to laugh as I snuffle my way through three quarters of a packet of Kleenex before the opening bars are even played.

There are more cameras than at an England press conference, with every parent eager to record these precious moments for posterity. But hark … from the distance we hear the sound of sobbing, first one child, then another, until 20 teary toddlers shuffle on to the stage to a rousing chorus of 'Rudolph the Red-nosed Reindeer'.

Our girl does better than most, getting to the fifth line of 'Twinkle Twinkle' before bawling her eyes out, but all we manage to catch on camera is a pair of fairy wings diving for the front row and the sanctuary of the parental lap.

Perhaps it is an omen. For this festive period turns out to be as wild as the last.

The child entertains everyone by telling them she is 'one and a half and a bit' and I entertain myself by training her to remove all the melamine and plastic ware from the dishwasher and 'put it cupboard'. Next step – dusting. Oh yes, we know how to rock and roll in this house.

Christmas Eve is a video of *Calendar Girls* and a box of Milk Tray. New Year's Eve, an early night.

But something mysterious has happened to our pump, so the boiler has packed up. And it's snowing outside. Just as we are about to freeze to death, at 3am the pilot light mysteriously and spontaneously ignites and the heating comes back on, clanking and spluttering. Then, at 5.07am, an errant helium balloon sets off the burglar alarm. At 5.39am, husband ends up in A&E with an ulcerated cornea.

Baby sleeps through the lot. Father spends the next 24 hours alternately daubing his eye with all manner of lotions and potions, and writhing around in agony. Mother starts the new decade a little weary and incapable of getting dressed.

Alas, the child does not really get the concept of a pyjama day, insisting it is a 'banana' day instead. I drink copious amounts of Diet Coke to try and wake myself up – before realising that it is caffeine free. And thus, as the day wears on, I get more tired and more grumpy by the minute.

While the child has her lunchtime nap, I log on to a social networking site to find a message from a 'home-schooling mom' who loves praise music and crystals and feels we must be 'good stewards to our temples'. She wants to know if I'm the Cari she was at school with. I am thinking that I'm not, although I do have a go at stewarding my temple with a curry and a bottle of wine, which feels pretty good to me and instantly makes the New Year a whole heap happier.

The dawning of another decade (and yes, there are pedants who are quite possibly right in insisting that the new decade actually begins at the start of 2011 and not 2010, but for the sake of argument, let's just go with it for now) has made me realise how quickly time flies.

It seems only moments ago that we were ushering in a new millennium (and no – please don't start with the whole 'technically that wasn't until 2001 … ') and yet 10 years have passed by in a flash, by which reckoning, the next time I blink I'll be a pensioner.

With this in mind, it seems prudent to make provision for the future, to ensure that the child will be well looked after in any eventuality. We put together wills and ponder over guardians, sadly accepting the fact that with grand-parents already in their 70s we'll have to look elsewhere.

A mum of a similar age confides, 'It makes me sad that my daughter won't get to know her grandparents as an adult.'

And when I realise that this will, most likely, be the case for my girl too it makes me pretty sad as well, especially when I think of the amazing bond I have continued to build with my own grandmothers well into my late 30s and mid-40s respectively.

But the situation is out of my hands. And other than continuing to ensure that the girl spends as much time as she can with her wider family, there is not a whole heap I can do about it – although it does make me all the more determined to cherish these precious relationships for as long as we possibly can.

The child is now 22 months old, and her latest fascination is bodily function. Until now, biology has not exactly been her strong point: 'Look, Mummy, there's a cow – milk comes out of its udder' (promising). Then, 'Look, Mummy, there's a sheep – milk comes out of its bottom' (oh). But I guess it's early days. She has begged us for a potty, and even though I am nowhere near ready to start toilet training (will I ever be?), I have relented.

Day One, and she wants to wander round the house with no nappy, vest unpopped and trailing behind her as she waltzes around her plastic throne.

I discover a puddle on the kitchen floor.

'Darling, you need to actually do it in … ' And then I see, she has! Yes, there is overspill, but the evidence of her prowess is there.

I am very proud (although I do fear for the shag pile rug if this continues). She, in turn, is very proud of her new undergarments and later in the afternoon is to be found at London Zoo, dress pulled over her head, shouting, 'Look, monkeys, I've got big-girl knickers and they're pink!'

The gorillas and the gibbons show not the blindest bit of interest, but undaunted she moves on to the ring-tailed lemurs, who are distinctly more approving.

However, she returns home rather damper of foot than is to be desired. So I 'accidentally' lose the potty while she is at nursery.

Nevertheless, a few days later I am impressed when she shouts out, 'Mummy, I need a wee.'

Then I see that she is clutching the mat we use as a 'magic carpet' and realise that what she actually means is, 'Mummy, I need a wheeeeee'. I guess it won't be long until it's, 'Mummy, I need a Wii'.

Indeed, 'I need' quickly becomes her favourite phrase: 'Mummy, I *need* a large croissant … Mummy, I *need* to go to the dentist and say, "Aaah" … Mummy, I *need* to go on an elloplane to America to build a campfire … '

Likewise, her earnest expression does its best to persuade me that she also 'needs' a 'Honey Cokey, right now', to 'wear swimming costume' (even though it is snowing outside) and 'to go to the zoo and see the animals. With a pink tissue' (sorry, love, white only and it's nursery today).

At bedtime, she stands up the minute I have left the room and calls, 'Mummy, I have woken up and I need to go in a submarine.' And when, at three in the morning, she insists she *needs* 'a piece of birthday cake and a balloon ride', I am almost tempted to give in, partly so I can stagger back to bed, but mainly because I feel guilty that I lied to her earlier in the day when she mistook my bag of Mini Eggs for acorns and I told her that yes, that was indeed what they were and therefore only squirrels could eat them.

I am a bad, bad mother – a fact that I can see that she herself is noting when she informs me she has banged her leg 'on a baby wipe' and I burst out laughing before I can stop myself. She looks at me with disdain and adds, 'very very badly, actually' before stomping off to seek more supportive solace from her bear.

I get my comeuppance, however, when an unfortunate incident involving a wooden giraffe results in considerable damage to my left knee. 'Humph,' says the starey, glarey look on the child's face. 'If you're looking to me for a bit of sympathy, you have come to the wrong place.'

And so, with a giraffine indentation attractively positioned at the point where the fake tan stops and the cellulite begins, I stagger to my feet to envelop her in the biggest hug I can muster.

'You know that I love you more than anything in the whole wide world?' I remind her.

'Humph,' she says. 'You forgot the universe.'

CHAPTER 9

TURNING TWO

The baby's second birthday is approaching. She is very much looking forward to the occasion and most nights can be heard singing, 'Happy Birthday' to herself in her cot. I am planning cakes (no surprise there, then); she is practising candle blowing, and has informed us that as her gift she would like 'yellow big-girl knickers and some Play-Doh'.

I am greatly cheered by the simplicity of her request, as I have realised that these days even the smallest of children seem to be such sophisticates that I am going to have enormous trouble in keeping up with the crowd.

When I was young we grew up slowly – we played with our Sindy horses until we hit double figures, then had a brief flirtation with pogo sticks and stilts, before graduating to the teenage grandeur of a Raleigh Twenty – or, if you were flash, a Shopper (which seemed to be exactly the same, but with a basket on the front).

Even birthdays were different then, in the era before PlayStations and Nintendo, when an 'apple' was something you gave the teacher at the end of term, rather than a byword for technological wizardry.

I remember very clearly the gifts that I got the day I turned 13, which included:

- 1 x Starsky and Hutch T-shirt (10 out of 10).
- 1 x black tracksuit with a yellow stripe down the side (9½ out of 10 – I clearly had no fashion sense).
- 1 x pink travel alarm clock in a hard round case that my grandmother would probably have dissed as being fuddy-duddy, yet which I believed to be the height of technological sophistication (9 out of 10).
- 1 x Hollie Hobbie beach set (floppy hat and matching frilled drawstring 'tote' bag) that I *actually used*. (At the time, I suspect that I may have given this a minimum of 8 out of 10, but hindsight is a powerful thing and embarrassment now only permits me to score in minus figures!).
- 1 x Silver Jubilee photo album – which, given it was now 1978 and said celebration had

taken place a year previous, seemed cheapskate
even to the unworldly child that I clearly was.

My parents bought me a tape recorder – and every Sunday
teatime, I would silence my younger siblings on pain of
death and lie on my bedroom floor, holding the plug-in
microphone against the side of the family radio in order to
record my favourite tunes from Radio One's chart
rundown. This was not as simple as it sounds, however, as
the phone seemed to ring every time I tried to 'capture'
anything by Brotherhood of Man, and I never did manage
to get a recording of Boney M's 'Rivers of Babylon' without Simon Bates talking over the beginning or the end.

As my own small girl's big day draws nearer I switch
into baking overdrive and she gets more excited by the
minute. I bake her a monkey cake for our family tea –
and it goes down a treat. Forget the scooter, the soft toys
and the many other generous gifts from relatives and
friends. When asked what she has been given, her reply
is always the same: 'A birthday balloon surprise and a
monkey cake with candles.'

I love that girl.

For her party, I attempt a Peppa Pig – easier than I
had imagined, though the red food colouring appears to
be indelible, and I am forced to explain to anyone who

catches sight of my hands that no, I am really not an axe murderer.

Together, we make biscuits for her friends and the house becomes a sea of sprinkles. The animal cupcakes are possibly a bridge too far – and as my husband is pressed into mini-marshmallow-chopping duty for the second year running, I do catch him muttering that I should just have gone to Tesco. But I am impervious to his discontent. I am swept away by my fantasies of being Nigella, Jane Asher and Annabel Karmel all rolled into one.

Yes, yes, I am the first to admit that my handiwork does not even come close to that of my culinary heroes. But it does make one little girl very happy. And frankly, that's all that matters.

Post party, and thanks in no small part to copious amounts of industrial-strength ibuprofen, life has returned to normal – or as normal as it can be in a household where a child apologises to her gingerbread man every time she takes a bite, and where conversation regularly heads along the following lines:

Me to child (for 10th time): Upstairs. NOW.
Her: No.

Me: Why not?

Her (in a convincingly caprine tone): Maaaah
  maaah.

Me: Eh?

Her: Because I am a goat, of course.

Or:

Me to child: Stop banging your cup on the table.

Her (looking pained and innocent): Oh Mummy,
  it's a donkey drumming its hoof beats to the
  dance.

I decide that it's time for a holiday.

Now the combination of an aversion to aviation (mine)
and a toddler who is unable to sit still for longer than 25
seconds (also mine) is possibly not entirely desirable
when it comes to planning and undertaking an excursion
overseas. And yet it would appear that the lure of
sunshine and abundant patisserie must have momentarily clouded any semblance of judgment and rationale that
I might otherwise have displayed, had I not been emerg-
ing pallid from the depths of an icy winter with an overwhelming craving for carbs and flaky pastry.

And thus, to celebrate the child's second birthday (quite brilliant timing, given that we now have to pay full whack for her), I find myself confirming a trip to the Continent, grappling with the mysteries of online check-in and purchasing an emergency set of bathroom scales in my panic that we might go a gramme over our allotted 15 kilos.

Until this point, we have not taken the child anywhere beyond a 200-mile radius of London, and the anticipation of her first trip in an 'elloplane' causes untold excitement (as witnessed by everyone who crosses our path in the build-up to the big day, including the dustman, the check-out lady in Tesco, a shifty-looking stranger hanging around near the park and the doctor who is doing her best to focus on the mechanics of performing my latest smear test).

'I go on a elloplane,' she trills to anyone who comes within a hundred yards. 'I sit down very carefully and put on my seat belt.'

I am somewhat dubious about the sitting-down part, recalling the London to Manchester train journey, during which it appeared that a magnetic field around her seat was preventing her from placing her behind anywhere close to it for the entire two hours.

And it is for this reason that at night I sneak into her room and whisper to her as she sleeps, hoping that somehow these subliminal messages will stop her rampaging around the plane and behaving in a way that I have always been able to tut at smugly in my child-free past. By day, I show her Googled images of the inside of an aircraft, complete with seated passengers in an effort to reinforce my point.

And so we arrive at the airport, deposit our baggage and attempt to restrain an overexcited toddler who is insisting on lying face-down on the floor in the centre of the departure lounge and becoming hysterical at any attempt to remove her.

She is no more enamoured of having to stand in the queue at the gate – and while my husband chases after her, I take the opportunity to suggest to our fellow passengers that it may be wise to select seats as far away from us as possible.

And yet, contrary to expectation, her behaviour on the flight is impeccable. True, she works out how to undo the seat belt within a nano second of sitting down, but I manage to convince her that the permanently lit 'No Smoking' sign actually means that you must keep your seat belt done up at all times – and remarkably, she falls for it hook, line and sinker.

With hindsight, I realise that it may have been a mistake to have read her a story about swashbuckling seafarers during the journey: as she voices her confusion between pirates and pilots I notice some consternation from the woman in front who is glancing nervously towards the cockpit and obviously wondering who's at the helm.

As recommended by a well-travelled friend, we are equipped with a variety of playthings to keep the child occupied and so we give her a sheet of stickers, most of which she adheres first to her top and then to my left arm – a fashion statement that does not go unnoticed by the rest of the passengers as we disembark.*

As the aircraft draws to a halt outside the terminal, the child takes it upon herself to befriend her fellow passengers with a rousing burst of 'Hello, everybody's to anyone and everyone within earshot, and then by clamping herself around the leg of the elderly French man who had been sitting innocently across the aisle and now finds

---

* It is only when I use the facilities before leaving the airport that I understand that the intense stares of the border guard at passport control were not, as I had thought, because I looked so much older and more haggard than in my (recent, but nicely coiffed) passport photo (this ageing almost entirely as a result of the earlier airport antics), but because I have a small yellow fish stuck firmly to the left of my nose.

himself bewildered by the attentions of a small girl trying to feed him the last of her raisins (and shouting, 'Howdy doody, nice to meet you, bye bye Cyril … ').

Fortunately, the airport is not a large one and so we are able to make it through to the car-hire desk without further incident – only to find that they have run out of the small (i.e. cheap) cars that we had booked, and so we have been upgraded to a vehicle that at first glance appears to be marginally longer than the *Ark Royal* and infinitely higher tech than my trusty Skoda back home. We waste half of the week trying to work out where the ignition and handbrake are, and most of the rest of it twiddling button after button in a vain attempt to open the windows.

Our holiday cottage is everything we had imagined and more: a rural idyll set in 16 acres of ponies, chickens, sheep and greenery, as far as the eye can see. As we ooh and aah over the surroundings, the child oohs and aahs over a plastic shopping basket full of plastic fruit and veg that she comes across the moment we enter and clutches for the entire seven days, refusing at any time to be separated from her 'cloud' – which could be plastic tomato slices or could be plastic jam (we never really do work it out).

For the first two days, we have the perfect holiday. The sun shines. The chickens lay eggs for our tea. My carb cravings are satisfied by a daily croissant delivery to our door.

Just as we are giving ourselves over entirely to the gods of relaxation and sloth, disaster strikes. It is first thing in the morning and the child has downed her morning milk and then fallen backwards and head first off our bed (high) and on to the floor (hard). She is shocked and screaming, but otherwise unresponsive and when she starts to vomit we panic and head for the nearest hospital (which is not very near at all).

In my best Franglais, I manage to establish that a) she is concussed, b) there is no paediatric department at this hospital and so we need to go to another one and c) that I really ought to have packed my dictionary.

An ambulance car transports me and the child, she drowsy and vomiting throughout the journey, me trying desperately to stop her from falling asleep and dabbing ineffectually at the mess with the one paper tissue the driver has to hand. Meanwhile, my husband follows in a car that is entirely unsuited to the winding country roads, and before we've even reached the halfway point one of the tyres has blown, and he is forced to abandon ship and join us for the rest of the journey.

By the time we arrive at hospital number two, the child is back on form, if a little whiffy, and after some

X rays, she is admitted for observation. Now my schoolgirl French may not be what it was (school being the best part of three decades ago), but even I am able to recognise the word 'grandmère' among a stream of questions that are thrown at me throughout the day. So now I get to be worried and depressed all at once, while entertaining a toddler without so much as a toy or a book to assist me in my task. I do lay my hands on a French maternity mag, and am delighted to find an article on the continental over 40s within – but without a dictionary, my understanding is somewhat sketchy and I don't get an awful lot further than 'old', 'old' and 'gestational diabetes'.

It is thanks in no small part to the owners of our cottage and only a microscopically small part to my linguistic abilities, that we arrive home that evening none the worse for our adventures and are able to enjoy the rest of our stay, despite the freezing rains which do not go especially well with the summer wardrobes that we packed in the spirit of optimism.

The return flight elicits as much excitement as the first, although once again, the toddler's airport antics are somewhat wearing. We have foolishly elected to head through passport control the minute we've checked in, not realising that the 'departure lounge' is actually the size of our own front room with a toilet in one corner and a vending machine in another. For two whole hours there is nothing to look at, nowhere to go, and, more importantly, nowhere to hide, as the child becomes bored with greeting our fellow passengers with, 'Hello lady, hello man, I'm a cheeky monkey' (mildly charming) and then announcing, 'I've done a dumpski and it's stinky' (less charming), before gradually losing the plot.

Taking her to the toilet with me seems like a good idea at the time, less so when she works out how to open the cubicle door while I am mid-flow and powerless to do anything but wave sheepishly to the people queueing outside.

It is no surprise that we find ourselves on the plane surrounded by empty seats – everyone else huddling as far away from us as they can at the back of the cabin. But some surprise that once again, the child is nothing short of angelic on the flight.

This time, she has spotted the safety information emblazoned on the back of the seat in front and wants to discuss it constantly and in depth throughout the journey – not necessarily an activity designed to appeal to the aviophobics among us. And so, while she and her father examine each picture in great detail, I feign sleep and do my best not to enlighten her with the reality:

'Daddy, why is the man climbing in the cupboard? Is he looking for a biscuit?'
(Actually, darling, he is throwing himself out of the emergency exit in order to avoid certain death.)
'Ooh – I would like a lovely yellow coat like that.'
(I would prefer that we do not have to try on the life jackets, if that's okay with you.)
'Can I go on the bouncy slide?'
(NO!)
'Look – the man is crawling. That's a nice game.'
(Yes – unless you notice that he is actually crawling through flames and smoke in a desperate but probably futile bid to flee a burning aircraft.)

Little wonder that it's good to get home.

And indeed, it is good to be home for a couple of days. Until, that is, an unwanted house guest in the form of chickenpox moves in for a fortnight, bringing with it several suitcases of extra washing and bearing a gift of a large bouquet of cabin fever.

To be fair, the child is an excellent patient bearing her affliction with great fortitude, relishing her antihistamine medication ('deee-licious, little bit more … ')

and reassuring us constantly that, 'I okay'. She accepts her imprisonment with good humour, while I climb the walls and spill calamine from a great height (and yes, still calamine – even after all these years).

At the end of her sentence, I take her to the doctor to be approved for her reintegration back into society. She is so excited to be out, to see a face other than ours, that she refuses to leave, lying on the floor outside the surgery, protesting violently at any attempt to prise her from the slightly threadbare carpet.

She is extricated only after much hysteria, consider-able brouhaha and extensive embarrassment, such that I can only hope that I stay fit and healthy for the foresee-able future, as I will not be able to show my face there again for at least another 15 years.

It is not the easiest trip home, given that pouring rain, a writhing and utterly incensed toddler in one arm and a buggy on the other do not necessarily make for easy passage. And thank you, passing stranger, for offer-ing biscuits, but I am holding strong against the bribery-to-avert-bad-behaviour movement. For now, at least. Although I admit that at times like this my resolve is being sorely tested …

*

Another day, another play date. Friends have come to tea, and although the children have been called to the table more than once, they are still dawdling and continuing their squabbles over who gets to hold the plastic teapot and who gets to brush the dolly's non-existent hair.

'Come along, girls, this won't get the baby a bonnet,' I urge, just as my mum always used to, while my mate regards me as though I have stepped straight from the planet Mars and asks me, 'What are you talking about and what would a baby be doing wearing a bonnet in any case – I thought it was only Jane Austen who went in for all that sort of nonsense.'

To make matters worse, the papers are full of Pixie Lott – a pop star of the noughties who, naturally, I have never heard of.

'I love all the old classic music,' she says. 'Bands like Take That, who my mum used to listen to.'

Given that I missed out on Take That first time round because I was too *old* (out of university, several years into my first job and way too much the working woman about town to be taking up with *boy* bands), it seems there is no hope. Why not lead me to my bath chair *now*?

This may be yet another reminder that I am an 'older mum', but I find consolation in the fact that I have met many, many others in exactly the same, slightly rickety, boat. And while I ask myself often what having an older mother may mean for my child, at least I know that I am not the only one to be grappling with such questions.

One friend reminds me: 'The bottom line (and one that the papers so often seem to forget) is that mother-hood is actually about far, far more than how old you happen to be when you have your child.'

And I agree. Kids need mums who are there for them and offer love, affection and support: if they can do that then frankly, it doesn't matter if they are 15 or 50 when they give birth. And if we're looking for positives, perhaps us older mums are less likely to resent our kids for ruining our figures/social lives/chances of becoming a pop star too. We know our limitations and are less likely to have false expectations of ourselves. (But hey – on the other hand, I've met older mums who've found having a child a terrible shock to the system; they were incredibly set in their ways and found the loss of independence appalling.)

In other words, as with anything else, it's horses for courses.

Perhaps I shall simply stick with the wise words of a former colleague: 'No matter what our age, there are two everlasting gifts we can give our children. One is roots, the other is wings.'

EPILOGUE

I am having a dream – it is a very nice dream, involving fluffy pillows, a stack of unread novels and a Nigella flourless chocolate cake – when suddenly I am aware of a dampness about my face. I assume initially that it is drool invoked by the sweet, sweet smell of the afore-mentioned patisserie, but it turns out to be the dribble of an enthusiastic toddler keen to involve me in her new favourite game of 'tooth fairies'.

'Look, Mummy,' she cries excitedly at the same time as shoving my head off the pillow with such vigour that I am forced to spend the rest of the day clutching a warmed wheat pillow to my aching neck for relief. 'The tooth fairy has left a coin.'

The 'coin', on this particular occasion, is played artfully by a tube of Germolene and will be used to buy crisps ('I must, must have some crisps, Mummy').

I have no idea where her fascination for potato chips has come from given that in her entire life she has consumed exactly two, long ago, at a party. And I am forced to refer my dear spouse to Section three, Subsection ii) of our lie-in treaty which clearly states that disturbance before 9am may only occur if a) it constitutes an extreme emergency or b) involves warmed croissants, strawberry conserve and freshly squeezed orange juice. I also have to remind him that Germolene has not been accepted as legal tender since we went decimal, and if he is insistent upon instructing the child in the art of pecuniary particulars he needs to pay a little more attention to detail.

And so it is that my first two years of motherhood draw to a close.

Two years in which I have enjoyed my daughter's company more than I could ever have imagined. In which I have told her a hundred times a day how much she is loved and how lucky I am to be her mum. In which I have discovered that all the clichés are actually true, and I would, indeed, scale the highest mountain or fight off lions bare-handed, if it meant I could protect her from harm.

That is not to say that I have been a perfect mother. Indeed if this is the time for confession let me hold up my hand, repent and say:

1) It was I who ate all the chocolate out of her party bags (and not a mouse).
2) Her yo yo is not mislaid. It is now in a land-fill site somewhere the other side of the North

Circular, having travelled there via our dust-
bin (though in my defence, I chucked it out
only because I thought she might strangle
herself with the string).

3) When I told her that she had to go straight
back to sleep because 'Mummy has a *lot* of
work to do', what I actually meant was that
Desperate Housewives was due to start in five
and I had forgotten to Sky-Plus it.

And that's before we take into account the whole list of
'things I swore I would never do, but seem to have actually done' (oops), which must be crowned by the birthday thank yous.

To elaborate further for the sake of clarity … For as
long as I can remember, I have been phobic about the
kind of missives of gratitude that run thus:

Dear Auntie Gladys
Thank you so much for your kind and generous gift
that you sent for my recent first birthday celebration.
It is very thoughtful and greatly appreciated and I
find all the brightly coloured shapes intensely stimu-
lating. I do hope that I will see you soon.
With love from Tallulah XXXXX

The very sight of such correspondence has always sent me all Victor Meldrew. And yet, and yet … in the wake of my daughter's recent birthday, I somehow find myself surrounded by letters purportedly written and signed by her.

What have I done? The girl is two. She cannot read or write. For heaven's sake, she only knows the letters M and P (which I realise does not make any literary endeavour on her part particularly easy, but is that really any excuse?).

Why did I do it? I, who have over the years lost count of the genius newborns who have thanked me for their 0–3 month Babygros in the most eloquent of manners, despite the fact they have only been on the earth for two weeks and haven't even learned to coo.

Would the donors of my daughter's birthday gifts not have been more charmed by an honest thank you from her mother, accompanied by an inarticulate scrawl – to add the personal touch – from the recipient herself?

I worry that my ill-advised forgery is only the beginning of a slippery slope that may see me abandon the rest of my principles before I know it. (If anyone catches me dressing the girl up like Bonnie Langford and parading her in front of friends and rellies with a cutesy song and dance act, shoot me please.)

Anyway … given that I may be deviating slightly, let us swiftly return to where we were before …

I have now been a mother, a mid-life mother, for two whole years – a period which has seen a lot of change:

- These days, though it pains me to admit it, I sport a not-so-nifty Caesarean overhang. And when I try to do the 'pencil test', I can now fit the whole of WH Smith's stationery department under my cleavage.
- I have bid farewell to a demanding but well-paid career.
- My house is no longer an homage to *Elle Decoration*, but filled instead with Stickle Bricks, soft toys and sticky fingermarks.
- Although I swore blind that my car would not end up like that of every other parent I have ever met (i.e. filled to the brim with crumbs, bits of broken breadstick, trodden-in raisins, manky soft toys and assorted other bits of child-related detritus), it is now *exactly* like that of every other parent I have ever met (i.e. filled to the brim with crumbs, bits of broken breadstick, trodden-in raisins, manky soft toys …).
- The social life that once consisted of premières and celebrity soirées is now made up of baby birthday parties and play dates in the park.
- Most of the time, I crave sleep in the way that an addict might crave alcohol or amphetamines.

But would I change a single thing? Not a chance.

I am the mother of the most delicious little girl on

the planet and there is nothing that could ever come close to beating that.

In reproductive terms, I may be pretty past it, but what better incentive to make sure I live and prosper for as long as I possibly can than a child who throws her arms around me saying, 'Mummy, let's have a little talk.'

'What shall we talk about, darling?'

'Fish.'

'Er, okay. Well, fish swim in the sea and they have—' (break off to comfort child who is now weeping).

'But, Mummy – what about the froggies?'

I am not sure I will ever be able to answer that one – nor, indeed, many others, including the reasoning behind the fact that she has recently taken to saying, 'Aaaah, poor poor Mummy', every time she gives me a hug. But what I do know is that I am very, very happy to be her geriatric mother, and I revel in every precious moment of parenthood.

Perhaps if you take away the cultural disparities, the odd grey hair and a fine set of bingo wings, being an older mum is really not so very different from being a younger mum. Day to day, it's certainly much the same: a squawking child is, after all, a squawking child, no matter how old you are when you are faced with one and have not the faintest idea of what's wrong.

And although all the over 40s I have spoken to say that they're permanently exhausted, most of the 20- and

30-somethings confess to being pretty shattered too. For whatever our age, we are all up to our eyes in nappies and nursery rhymes. We all share the same sleepless nights worrying about shrinking catchment areas and how to get tomato pasta out of our dry-clean-only trousers.

And although the number of mid-life mums continues to rise, and in many parts of the country, indeed the world, it becomes ever more the norm, what people seem to forget is that it's really not that new for women to be giving birth when they're 'past their prime'. As one friend (kids at 40 and 46) says:

'I really have no idea about why the media continue to make such a fuss about the whole thing. We live near Darwin's house in Downe, Kent and we visited it while I was pregnant. Upstairs, they have a family tree on one wall and you can see that even way back then, the women were producing children – with only the assistance of Mother Nature – well into their 40s. Older than me in fact. Hurrah.'

Yes, we have seen that there are advantages to being an older mum – and yes, of course, we have seen that there's a flip side too, as there is, indeed, with everything in life (except, possibly, Häagen-Dazs Cookies & Cream).

Some older mums have found it hard to accept that after all these years the established pattern of their lives has changed ('I don't have as much patience as I thought I would. I am set in my ways in so many respects and have had to learn that I cannot always be in total control – not easy!').

For others, giving birth and witnessing the miracle of life has made them question their own mortality. 'It upsets me a lot that if my daughter has her children as late as me I might not live to see them.'

It's a theme that is echoed by many. And asking around uncovers a whole list of other concerns. Will we be mistaken for grandmothers at the school gates? Will we have forgotten what it's like to be a teenager by the time our kids reach that stage? How will we deal with pubescent outbursts if we're struggling with the menopause ourselves? (As a close friend says, 'That's one hell of a lot of hormones to fit in one small semi!')

As for me? Yes, I worry about all these things and more. But hey – I'm certain I'll cope. Sure, there may be a decade between me and many of the other new mums I meet, but they say you are as old as you feel.

In my case, that's usually around 107. But I've discovered it takes just one cheeky grin, one, 'Love you, Mummy,' from my beloved girl to put a youthful spring in my step. So should you be wandering around my neighbourhood, at least when the weather warms up a bit, you may just catch me casting off the support stockings and dancing in the street like a young 'un.

ACKNOWLEDGEMENTS

A huge thank you to the following:

- Spencer Debson, whose Facebook comment started this whole ball rolling.
- The *JC*, especially Stephen Pollard, for giving me the column and for allowing me to use the material in this book.
- Andrew Prentice, for his expert medical advice.
- Gaye Henson and Heulwen Morgan for their care, calm and patience.
- My friends, for being on the end of a phone 24/7 at the beginning when I didn't have a clue what I was doing, and for the generous loan of baby paraphernalia, clothes and toys galore.
- The many fantastic women who have helped me with my research by sharing their own stories and experiences.

- Jonathan Pegg – partly because I have always wanted the chance to be able to say 'my agent', but mainly because without him this wouldn't have happened.

- Susanna Abbott and Miranda West at Vermilion, for giving me the chance to write this book and for making it such an enjoyable journey. Also to Gill Paul for her editorial wisdom and Lucy Stephens for the fantastic cover design.

- Mum, Dad, Kiah and the rest of my lovely family, for far too many things to mention individually.

- My husband Rob for his unfailing love, support and encouragement (and for doing all the washing).

And most of all – thank you to the little girl who inspired this book. You make my heart sing and bring me more joy than I could ever have imagined.